Employment Issues and
MULTIPLE SCLEROSIS

D1227440

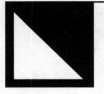

Employment Issues and

MULTIPLE SCLEROSIS

Second Edition

Phillip D. Rumrill, Jr.
Kent State University
Center for Disability Studies
Kent, Ohio

Mary L. Hennessey
University of Florida
Department of Behavioral Science
and Community Health
Gainsville, Florida

Steven W. Nissen
National Multiple Sclerosis Society
National Capital Chapter
Washington, DC

With invited contributions

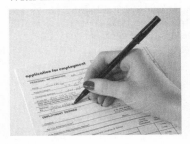

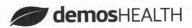

Visit our website at www.demosmedpub.com

Library of Congress Cataloging-in-Publication Data

Employment issues and multiple sclerosis / Phillip D. Rumrill Jr., Mary L. Hennessey, Steven W. Nissen ; with invited contributors. — 2nd ed.
    p. ; cm.
Includes bibliographical references and index.
ISBN-13: 978-1-932603-64-4 (pbk. : alk. paper)
ISBN-10: 1-932603-64-6 (pbk. : alk. paper)
    1. Multiple sclerosis—Patients—Employment—United States. I. Hennessey, Mary L. II. Nissen, Steven W. III. Rumrill, Phillip D.
[DNLM: 1. Multiple Sclerosis—United States. 2. Disabled Persons—legislation & jurisprudence—United States. 3. Employment—legislation & jurisprudence—United States. 4. Rehabilitation, Vocational—United States. WL 360 R937e 2008]
RC377.R85 2008
362.196'834—dc22

                                    2007047859

SPECIAL DISCOUNTS ON BULK QUANTITIES of Demos Medical Publishing books are available to corporations, professional associations, pharmaceutical companies, health care organizations, and other qualifying groups. For details, please contact:

Special Sales Department
Demos Medical Publishing
386 Park Avenue South, Suite 301
New York, NY 10016
Phone: 800–532–8663 or 212–683–0072
Fax: 212–683–0118
Email: orderdept@demosmedpub.com
Made in the United States of America
07 08 09 10   5 4 3 2 1

For Harry, Beverly, Stuart, Douglas, and Nathan
—PDR

For Megan, Matthew, Zachary, Mitchell, and Samuel
—MLH

For Mom, Dad, and Max
—SWN

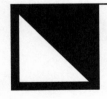

Contents

Preface

MULTIPLE SCLEROSIS (MS) is one of the most common neurological disorders in the Western Hemisphere. It affects as many as half a million people in the United States alone. Experts in the medical and social sciences have documented the wide-ranging effects that MS exacts on a person's physical, psychological, and social functioning, and virtually every aspect of life has proven susceptible to the illness. The barriers to employment and career development posed by MS render the illness even more debilitating than the medical symptoms themselves. Although the vast majority of people with MS have employment histories and were working at the time of diagnosis, many are unable to maintain employment as the illness progresses. This deprives society of a well-trained, experienced, and productive labor resource, so more focused efforts are needed to help more people with MS stay in the work force as long as they wish to.

Like its first edition, *Employment Issues and Multiple Sclerosis*, which was published in 1996, this second edition focuses on the employment issues that people with MS face as they cope with a highly unpredictable and sometimes severe chronic illness. This second edition represents a 30 to 35 percent revision of the first volume, and all information that was presented in the original volume has been updated to reflect the current state of research, legislation, policy, and service delivery. The nine chapters in this edition address (a) an overview of the medical and psychosocial aspects of MS, (b) factors associated with employment status among people with MS, (c) vocational assessment strategies for people with MS, (d) vocational interventions for people with MS, (e) the Americans with Disabilities Act, (f) the Family and Medical Leave Act and the Health Insurance Portability and Accountability Act, (g) Social Security disability programs, (h) a perspective on employment from the National Multiple Sclerosis Society, and (j) recommendations to improve the employment opportunities and outcomes of people with MS.

The first four chapters present research-based and somewhat technical descriptions of the medical, psychosocial, and vocational aspects of MS. Specialized terms and professional jargon are defined in text. With those foundations established, the remaining five chapters are devoted to "plain English" discussions of federal legislation, government programs, advocacy efforts, and other resources that provide employment-related supports and services for people with MS.

Intended for people with MS, their friends and families, physicians, nurses, social workers, disability advocates, allied health practitioners, counselors, psychologists, employers, human resource managers, rehabilitation professionals, and anyone else interested in the employment implications of MS, the second edition of *Employment Issues and Multiple Sclerosis* is a resource guide to matters of research, public policy, and service delivery. The text also discusses current trends in health care and rehabilitation and recommends reforms to better serve the interests of people with MS.

Phillip D. Rumrill, Jr., PhD, CRC
Mary L. Hennessey, PhD, CRC
Steven W. Nissen, MS, CRC

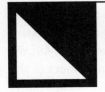

Acknowledgments

W E WOULD LIKE TO take this opportunity to thank our friends and colleagues throughout the United States who guided and assisted us in the development of this, the second edition of *Employment Issues and Multiple Sclerosis*. Their inspiration, expertise, support, and encouragement were instrumental to our efforts to complete this project, and we could not have done this without them.

First, we thank the outstanding editorial staff at Demos Medical Publishing for the opportunity to publish this work, for their editorial consultation, and for their technical assistance. We look forward to other collaborative ventures with Demos Medical Publishing in the future.

Our gratitude goes to Kimberly Calder of the National Multiple Sclerosis Society, who contributed an excellent chapter (Chapter 6) on continuation of health insurance benefits, health insurance portability, and unpaid family and medical leave. We also wish to thank Dr. Richard Roessler of the University of Arkansas for contributing an excellent chapter (Chapter 3) on vocational assessment, and we gratefully acknowledge all of Dr. Roessler's research and program development efforts to promote employment opportunities for Americans with multiple sclerosis (MS).

We are also grateful to Dr. Nicholas LaRocca of the National Multiple Sclerosis Society for his pioneering research and advocacy efforts regarding the employment of people with MS, as well as for his generous support of our research programs over the years.

The National Multiple Sclerosis Society has a long and successful tradition of employment services and programs for people with MS. We want to acknowledge past and present professional staff members of the Society who have helped thousands of Americans with MS seek, secure, and maintain employment: Dr. Beverly Noyes, Diane Afes, Carolyn Konnert, Kincaid Early, Greg Kovach, Beth Robertson, Michelle Jones, Jill Zorn, Judy Cotton, Pete Kennedy, Nancy Law, Melissa Roby, Debbie Rios, Kent Wiles, Becky Wiehe, Susan Raimondo, Gary Sumner, John Carnesecchi, Barbara McKeon, Pam Hirshberg, Karen Mariner, Mike Van Abel, and Mary Elizabeth McNary. We also wish to thank all of the chapters of the Society and the individuals with MS who have participated in our research and community service projects over the past two decades.

We are indebted to our fellow researchers and scholars who have collaborated with us in research related to employment and MS, provided us with opportunities to publish our work in this area, and inspired us through their own research and writing on the subject. These friends and esteemed colleagues include Drs. Rosalind Kalb, Robert Fraser, Nicholas LaRocca, Bryan Cook, Lynn Koch, Brian McMahon, Shawn Fitzgerald, Karen Jacobs, Paul Wehman, Richard Roessler, Jeanne Neath, George Denny, Courtney Viestra, Darlene Unger, Joanne Gottcent, and Gary Sumner.

For their clerical, editorial, and research assistance in completing this text, we thank Joseph Carroll, Suzanne Savickas, Elizabeth Omar, Linnea Carlson, and Jodi Swan—all of the Kent State University Center for Disability Studies. Their watchful eyes, careful pens, and accurate reference checks made it possible for us to deliver a clean and well-formatted manuscript to the publisher in a timely fashion.

Finally, and most especially, we extend our deep appreciation, gratitude, and respect to people with MS, their friends, and their significant others who work so courageously and so persistently to combat the devastating effects that MS can have in virtually every aspect of life. The incredible contributions that these individuals continue to make to society while coping with such an unpredictable and intrusive disease humble and inspire us, and it is both a pleasure and a privilege for us to work with this truly remarkable group of people.

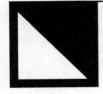

Contributors

Kimberly Calder, MPS
Senior Manager, Insurance Initiatives
National Multiple Sclerosis Society
New York, New York

Mary L. Hennessey, PhD, CRC
Assistant Professor of Rehabilitation Counseling
Department of Behavioral Science and Community Health
University of Florida
Gainesville, Florida

Steven W. Nissen, MS, CRC
Director of Employment Programs
National Multiple Sclerosis Society
National Capital Chapter
Washington, DC

Richard T. Roessler, PhD, CRC
University Professor of Rehabilitation Education & Research
University of Arkansas
Fayetteville, Arkansas

Phillip D. Rumrill, Jr., PhD, CRC
Professor of Rehabilitation Counseling
Director, Center for Disability Studies
Kent State University
Kent, Ohio

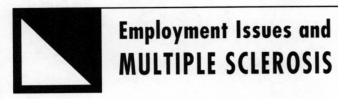

Employment Issues and
MULTIPLE SCLEROSIS

Overview of Multiple Sclerosis

Mary L. Hennessey

Phillip D. Rumrill, Jr.

I N THIS CHAPTER, we provide an overview of multiple sclerosis (MS), one of the most prevalent and unpredictable neurological disorders in the world. We will begin with a description of how MS manifests itself in the brain and along the spinal cord, and then follow with discussions of the history of the disease, risk factors, causes, courses and progression, diagnosis, physiological effects, psychological effects, and treatment. The intent of this chapter is to introduce the reader to the disease and how it affects people; much of the material presented in summary form in this chapter will be examined at greater length in terms of the impact of the disease on employment in subsequent chapters.

What Is MS?

MS is one of the most common neurological diseases known to medical science. It is a degenerative disease of the central nervous system, primarily affecting the brain and the spinal cord. MS destroys the fatty tissue, called myelin, that surrounds white matter tracts (i.e., axons) in multiple locations in the brain and along the spinal cord. The purpose of the myelin is to facilitate the axons' conduction of electrical impulses back and forth from the brain to the rest of the body via the spinal cord (1,2). In areas where the myelin is destroyed or compromised, these electrical impulses, which coordinate all mental and physiological processes, are not conveyed as they should be. This slowed or blocked conduction of information can have a disruptive influence on virtually every physical, sensory, mental, and emotional activity.

Smith and Schapiro (3) described the demyelination that occurs in MS as similar to the disruption of an impulse or message that would occur if the rubberized coating surrounding a telephone or electrical wires were torn or cut. Such damage interferes with the transmission of information and/or electricity, which is precisely what happens in individuals with MS. For people with MS, the result is often observed as uncoordinated and/or awkward responses to environmental stimuli (2). As patches of myelin deteriorate, they are replaced by scar tissue. The resulting lesions, or plaques, further interrupt the conduction of nerve impulses, sometimes creating a progressive and degenerative course of symptoms.

Symptoms associated with MS vary widely depending upon the location and size of the lesions in the person's brain and spinal cord (2,4). For example, frontal and parietal lobe lesions often result in cognitive and emotional effects, whereas plaques in the cerebrum, brain stem, and spinal cord tend to cause problems related to the physical functioning of the extremities (1,5). Visual impairments may result from direct damage to the optic nerves or the occipital lobe. A significant impediment to fully understanding the etiology of MS lies in the fact that no two people with MS experience the same symptoms and course of illness (6). Existing research on the physiological and psychological symptoms of MS is described in greater detail in subsequent sections of this chapter. For additional information concerning the medical aspects of MS, readers are referred to other texts (1,2,7–9).

History, Risk Factors, and Causes

Medical historians speculate that MS was first observed as far back as the fourteenth century, but the documented history of the disease began in the nineteenth century with the first clinical descriptions and illustrations surfacing during the 1820s and 1830s (1,2,10). In 1824, the first patients were diagnosed with symptoms that would today definitively characterize MS. These diagnoses appeared in the diary of Auguste D'Estes, which also included a personal account of his own experiences with what would now be know as optic neuritis and relapsing-remitting MS (10). Despite these clinical observations, MS was not given a name until 1868, when the French physician Jean-Martin Charcot labeled it

"Sclerose en Plaques." Charcot is recognized as the first scientist to link the symptoms of MS to demyelination and lesions in the central nervous system (9,11). In the next century, medical science made steady progress in the quest to understand the etiology of MS and to ameliorate its effects. Most notable among these efforts were the 1921 meeting of the Association of Research in Nervous and Mental Disease, the work of Russell Brain in the 1930s, a comprehensive monograph on the medical aspects of MS written by McAlpine et al. (12), and the continual search for and refinement of chemotherapeutic strategies to treat MS beginning in the 1970s (9,11).

Moving ahead to 2007, MS is well established as one of the most common neurological disorders in the Western Hemisphere. The National Multiple Sclerosis Society (NMSS) estimates the prevalence of MS in the United States to be between 350,000 and 400,000 cases, indicating that 1 in 750 people have the diagnosis at any given time (1,3). It has been estimated that 10,000 new cases of MS are diagnosed each year in the United States, and this rate of incidence has steadily increased since the 1950s. This heightened rate of detection has been attributed to the advent and refinement of increasingly sensitive diagnostic tools such as magnetic resonance imaging (13). In a worldwide study, Dean (14) determined that approximately 1,080,000 people across the globe have MS (i.e., 20.6 cases per 100,000 people).

Although MS can occur at any age, initial manifestations are most often evident during early adulthood, typically between the ages of 20 and 40 (2,5,8). In fact, half of MS diagnoses are conferred before the person's 30th birthday, and three-quarters of Americans with MS were diagnosed before the age of 40 (1,15).

MS is diagnosed much more frequently among women than men. MS is approximately two to three times more common in women than in men, a gender propensity that is found in a host of other autoimmune diseases (1,16). The prevalence of MS also varies markedly according to geography. Epidemiological studies have revealed higher MS prevalence rates in temperate regions than in warmer climates. Countries that have particularly high rates of MS include the United Kingdom, Canada, Germany, Denmark, Norway, Sweden, Finland, and the United States (3,17). Within the United States, epidemiologists have cited the 37th parallel (which divides the American population roughly in half) as a geographical demarcation that separates areas marked by high and low MS risks (18). Two-thirds of the American MS population resides in the northernmost 50 percent of the general populace, with the states of Vermont and Washington reporting the highest prevalence rates in the United States (1,2).

The incidence and prevalence of MS vary significantly along racial lines, as well. Poser (19) pointed out that MS is extremely uncommon among Asian peoples, unknown in African blacks, and relatively infrequent among African Americans. He also noted that people of Hispanic descent are far less likely to develop MS than those of Germanic, Anglo-Saxon, and Scandinavian lineages. More recent studies of the racial and ethnic characteristics of people with MS have yielded similar findings (3).

For all of the research that has been conducted to gain a better understanding of this complicated disease, the precise cause of MS remains unknown. That said, experts believe that MS stems from a combination of immunological, viral, and genetic factors. Although studies show that certain groups (e.g., women, people of Northern European descent, people living in the Northern Hemisphere) are more likely to acquire MS than others, how and why MS originates in an individual remains less certain. Medical scientists have determined that MS involves an autoimmune process; that is, the immune system abnormally directs itself against the central nervous system. Although the exact antigen to which immune cells are directed has not been identified, researchers have discovered which immune cells become sensitized, the process by which they turn on the central nervous system, and which receptors on the cells are attracted to the myelin sheath (8).

Epidemiological studies and migration patterns indicate that people who were born in regions where there is a high prevalence of MS and who move to lower prevalence areas acquire the MS risk of their new homes, provided that the move takes place before the age of 15 (17). From these data, some scientists have inferred that there is an environmental agent which activates prior to puberty and predisposes one to develop MS in early or middle adulthood. Because initial exposure to many viruses occurs during childhood, and because viral factors have been linked to many other demyelinating autoimmune responses, some experts believe that viral "triggers" precipitate the onset of the illness.

Although MS is not hereditary, having a first-degree relative (e.g., a parent or sibling) who has the illness increases one's risk of acquiring MS by a factor several times that of the risk in the general population (3,6). Being the daughter of a person with MS makes one 10 times more likely than the general population to acquire the disease during adulthood (1). Several studies have also found common genes among certain populations in which there are high rates of MS. The HLA gene group is where some of the genes linked to MS have been found (1); however efforts to isolate a single "MS gene" have proven unfruitful. Some neurologists and epidemiologists hypothesize that MS develops when a person is genetically susceptible to environmental agents or factors (including viruses) that trigger autoimmune responses (1). That explanation assumes a reciprocal influence of immunological, viral, and genetic factors in the development of MS, but its complexity underscores why pinpointing the illness' precise cause remains an elusive pursuit.

Courses and Progression

Whether someone's experience with multiple sclerosis is in a personal or professional context, he or she realizes that the unpredictable disease process is one of the most problematic aspects of the disorder. Certainly, the nature, severity, and number of symptoms related to MS vary widely among individuals. Moreover, the patterns of symptom manifestation, which are typically observed in terms of relapses and remissions, cannot be generalized from one person to the next; as mentioned earlier in this chapter, no two people with MS experience the exact same disease process. These patterns have, however, been broadly codified to provide a clearer understanding of the different types of MS that people experience.

Current classification standards in the field of neurology describe four types or courses of MS: (a) relapsing-remitting, (b) primary progressive, (c) secondary progressive, and (d) progressive relapsing (1,2,10,16). The characteristic patterns of each course of MS follow.

Relapsing-Remitting MS

Smith and Schapiro (3) described relapsing-remitting MS as being marked by clearly defined flare-ups (also called relapses, exacerbations, or attacks) that begin at the onset of the disease and last from days to weeks, with or without asymptomatic periods. These flare-ups are episodes of acute worsening in neurological functioning and they may be totally unpredictable. They are followed by recovery periods (remissions), which are either partial or complete. Fraser et al. (1) stated these sporadic exacerbations occur at an average rate of approximately one time every 17 months. Disability may result from incomplete recoveries following relapse, but relapses tend not to become progressively severe or intense

5

over time. Schapiro (2) noted that about 80 percent of MS cases begin as relapsing-remitting MS, making it far and away the most common form of the disease at the time of diagnosis.

Primary Progressive MS

Primary progressive MS is observed when the person evinces a slow but steady decline in functioning from the onset of the disease. In this course, there do not appear to be noticeable relapses or remissions (16). If a person does experience a plateau, it is temporary and improvement in symptoms is minor. Primary progressive MS is commonly diagnosed in people who develop the disease after their 40th birthday (2), and this group makes up about 10 percent of the MS population with equal ratios of females to males (1).

Secondary Progressive MS

Secondary progressive MS is characterized by initial relapsing-remitting MS which subsequently develops into a steady progressive course, with or without flare-ups, remissions, or plateaus (10,16). Over time, secondary progressive MS results in a decline in the person's general health status, while exacerbations become less frequent (1). It is estimated that about two-thirds of people diagnosed with relapsing-remitting MS eventually develop the secondary progressive form of the disease (1). Currently, physicians are not able to predict who will develop secondary progressive MS based on the initial onset of the disease (3).

Progressive Relapsing MS

In progressive relapsing MS, affected people experience a steady and progressive course of declining health over time, but they also have clear and significant exacerbations or relapses that occur without warning (16). Symptoms are always present, but they may intensify or decrease in severity from time to time (2). Coupled with the steady progression of symptoms, this cycle of exacerbation can be truly debilitating. This type of MS is relatively rare and occurs in approximately 5 percent of cases (16).

Diagnosis

Until fairly recently, the diagnosis of MS was inferred from presenting symptoms as there is no genetic, bacterial, or viral test that can make the diagnosis (1). Because central nervous system lesions can result from conditions other than MS (such as cancer, nutritional deficiencies, or traumatic brain injuries), neurologists would first eliminate all other possible reasons for lesions before making a diagnosis of MS. Hence, the differential diagnostic process was often long and laborious (5). Not surprisingly, nondiagnoses and misdiagnoses were fairly common, and many patients were sent home with "possible" and "probable" MS to wait for their symptoms to progress before they could receive definitive diagnoses. Needless to say, this waiting exacted a significant psychological toll on patients and their families (20).

Over the past two decades, however, the advent and continued refinement of magnetic resonance imaging (MRI) and positron emission tomography (PET) have enabled neurologists to make accurate MS diagnoses in a timely manner, sometimes even before the person evinces any symptoms (5). The current standard criteria used to diagnose MS are known as McDonald criteria (1,2). These criteria require multiple abnormalities on MRI and PET scans in the central nervous system (CNS). In descending order of prevalence, the CNS abnormalities observed in people with MS affect the following functional areas: sensation and energy, vision, strength and mobility, coordination, balance, bowel and bladder processes, sexuality, cognition, and affect and emotion. Although these criteria permit diagnosis before people have experienced MS-related symptoms, this is not common because it is the symptoms of MS that prompt people to seek medical attention in the first place.

The MRI and PET scans have also shown promise in predicting the frequency, duration, and intensity of exacerbations of MS following diagnosis (9). Even though not all symptoms of MS reported in clinical consultation are directly attributable to MRI and PET scan abnormalities, neurologists are able to make MS diagnoses with greater speed and accuracy than ever before. Medical technology has dramatically reduced the time interval between initial symptoms and diagnosis, thereby enabling rehabilitation professionals to initiate early intervention strategies during the disease's preliminary stages. That said, medical technology is no substitute for the clinical judgment of physicians who must first observe possible or probable MS symptoms and then choose the appropriate diagnostic protocol. No matter the protocol or diagnostic criteria used, a diagnosis of MS requires damage to the central nervous system in more than one place, evidence of multiple damage at more than one point in time, and elimination of alternative explanations for the damage (8,10).

Physiological Effects

The constellation of physiological symptoms of MS extends over a wide range, including fatigue, mobility problems, spasticity, numbness and tingling in the extremities, general weakness, visual impairments, bowel and bladder dysfunction, and sexual dysfunction. As previously noted, patterns of symptoms have been attributed to the location and size of lesions in the central nervous system and are specific to the individual (1). Even within the individual with MS, physiological and other effects may come and go without warning, appear in various combinations, or intensify in a seemingly random pattern (13). Any physiological symptoms of MS may be observed in concert with or in the absence of any other(s). The wide range of physical symptoms and the capricious disease process pose significant impediments for people with MS in virtually every aspect of personal and social functioning.

Fatigue

The most common effect of MS is unquestionably fatigue (2,8). Fatigue has been defined as an overwhelming sense of tiredness, lack of energy, and feelings of exhaustion in excess of what might be expected for the associated level of activity (9). Although it does not always present itself as a single, easily identifiable symptom, fatigue affects people with MS in several specific ways. Schapiro (2) identified three distinct types of fatigue that are commonly observed in people with MS: *deconditioned, "short-circuiting,"* and *MS fatigue*. Each has unique signs and self-care implications.

DECONDITIONED FATIGUE. When people with MS experience weakness, heat sensitivity, and fatigue, they may become less active over time. This lack of activity creates a vicious cycle, in which they become even weaker and more tired (3). Over time, the body becomes deconditioned to physical activity, muscle can atrophy, and secondary complications of inactivity often manifest themselves. These secondary complications include weight gain, hypertension and other circulatory problems, arthritis, and heart disease. When noticed early in the disease process, deconditioned fatigue can be alleviated by an overall wellness program that includes individualized exercise and nutrition plans.

SHORT-CIRCUITING. According to Schapiro (2), short-circuiting fatigue or muscle fatigue results from physically overtaxing oneself.

He noted that demylination along neural pathways leads to interruptions in the smooth transmission of electrical impulses to the extremities. This inefficiency results in temporary weakness of the limbs, which then produces the slowing and eventual stoppage of physical activity until people with MS have rested and regained their energy. Short-circuiting fatigue is primarily physiological in nature, and stopping activity to allow the nerves and muscles to restart is the way to manage this form of fatigue (3). Unlike deconditioned fatigue, which is often progressive in nature and can result in permanent debilitation, short-circuiting fatigue is temporary, episodic, and managed fairly effectively by rest and relaxation.

MS FATIGUE. Smith and Schapiro (3) describe lassitude as MS fatigue because it seems to be endemic to people coping with the illness. MS fatigue is typified by an overwhelming sense of exhaustion or tiredness that affects the individual suddenly and without warning. These bouts of complete, physiological, and psychological tiredness and incapacity may last for a few hours, or they may extend for several days. Some people report that relaxation or rest mitigates these symptoms, but others have reported these solutions do not work for them. Lassitude of this type usually responds to neurochemical medications, and also an individualized aerobic exercise program (3). They also aptly noted that MS fatigue is linked, often bidirectionally, to medication side effects, depression, and sleep disturbances.

Generally, all types of fatigue that are commonly reported by people with MS are exacerbated by stress and by an increase in body temperature. Because exercise, being outside in hot weather, and taking hot baths have been shown to increase fatigue among people with MS, these activities should be monitored or avoided whenever possible. Also, stress management regimens have proven to be effective means of controlling fatigue and allowing the person with MS to conserve energy for necessary daily living activities.

Motor Disturbances

A number of physiological symptoms are related to motor disturbances in people with MS, including spasticity, weakness, and ataxia. These lead to general coordination, balance, and mobility impairments (2,8). The extent and type of these effects vary widely among (and even within) people with MS, but motor disturbances are typically among the first manifestations of the illness.

SPASTICITY. Spasticity is a disruption in the coordination of muscle contraction and relaxation. This is a common symptom of MS because of damage in the descending motor pathways that carry impulses from the spinal cord to control muscular reflexes. When lesions occur along these pathways, they cause opposite muscles within a group to contract and relax simultaneously, or spasm. Spasms are most common in the legs (flexor and extensor muscles), and people with MS most frequently experience spasticity at night (3,8).

WEAKNESS. MS is often characterized by a loss of strength in major muscle groups such as those of the arms and legs. Smith and Schapiro (3) noted that observed weakness in people with MS more often results from poorly transmitted neural impulses than from deterioration of the muscles themselves. However, misconduction of impulses makes it difficult for the person with MS to fully utilize the affected muscles, and prolonged underutilization can cause the muscles to atrophy.

Backaches are a common secondary symptom of MS, most often attributable to strain resulting from compensation for weakness and fatigue in the legs (2). Ataxia, one's inability to move the arms and walk in a coordinated fashion, is another frequently observed effect of MS-related weakness.

In combating muscular weakness, priority must be placed on conserving energy for activities of daily living and symptom management. Because some exercises exacerbate muscle weakness and fatigue, people with MS should always consult their physicians and/or physical therapists before initiating a physical conditioning program.

AMBULATION. Ambulation, the simple act of walking and getting around, is often impaired by such symptoms of MS as balance problems, hyperextension of the knees, and instability of the legs. A condition called *foot drop* (2), in which toes touch the ground prior to the heel is caused by weak muscles in the foot. Ambulation problems in people with MS can range from mild difficulties to a complete inability to stand or walk on one's own. Canes, motorized scooters, and other mobility aides are often employed by people with MS who experience difficulty with ambulation.

Numbness and Tingling

Numbness and tingling in the extremities among people with MS can range from "pins and needles" sensations to itching in an isolated area of skin or a more severe and painful condition termed *trigeminal neuralgia* (3). A pins and needles sensation down the back and legs may occur when the neck is bent. Although not painful, the sensation can be bothersome. Trigeminal neuralgia involves the onset of sudden, sharp pain in one side of the face. It results from the discharge of impulses from the brain stem. The accompanying pain typically lasts for only 10 to 15 seconds, but it is characteristically followed by a facial contraction, or tic (8).

Tremor

Tremor in the extremities and head is another common physiological effect of MS, one that is manifested in a wide range of movement from fine, less noticeable tremors to more obvious, gross oscillations (2). Tremors occur in approximately 75 percent of people with MS and most often are seen in the upper limbs. They can be significantly disabling, affecting limb function, gait, and balance (9). Functionally speaking, tremors can have a deleterious impact on common work-related fine motor tasks such as writing, keyboarding, and handling small objects.

Visual Impairments

Visual impairments in individuals with MS are most often temporary conditions that manifest in blurred or double vision, although, in some cases, functional blindness may result. They result from optic neuritis (i.e., inflammation of the optic nerve) and are frequently marked by dull color vision, diminished visual acuity, and a reduced visual field (2). Optic neuritis is one of the most common early symptoms of MS (2,10), and it is often indicative of a more benign form of the illness. Other MS-related visual impairments result from weakening of the eye muscle and nystagmus (i.e., eye jerking). MS-related visual impairments often lead to a diminished ability to drive or travel independently, which can cause major difficulties in terms of employment and community living.

Bowel and Bladder Dysfunction

Bowel and bladder dysfunction are frequent, frustrating, and often embarrassing effects of MS. Polman et al. (9) indicated that some degree of bladder dysfunction occurs in at least 70 percent of those diagnosed with MS, and up to two-thirds of all people with MS complain of some degree of bowel dysfunction. These difficulties include urgency, dribbling, hesitancy, frequency, constipation, and incontinence. Bowel and bladder dysfunctions can have a negative impact on a person's daily living regimen, but they often can be effectively managed through medications and/or diet.

Sexual Dysfunction

Sexual dysfunction affects up to 85 percent of men and up to 74 percent of women diagnosed with MS (21). The issue of sexual dysfunction in people with MS requires close consideration within the context of general symptomatology. The effects of sexual dysfunction can be pervasive, often manifesting in psychological and family problems in addition to their physiological accompaniments. Often associated with fatigue, specific sexual problems frequently encountered by people with MS include retarded and premature ejaculation, decreased vaginal and penile sensation, impotence, vaginal dryness, anorgasmia, decreased sex drive, and slowed response and arousal time (9).

Psychological Effects

As if the physiological accompaniments of MS were not debilitating enough, the illness often has a negative impact on one's psychological functioning. Psychological problems related to MS can be divided into three categories: (a) cognitive dysfunction, (b) affective disorders, and (c) adjustmental issues. Texts by Kalb (7) and Frazer et al. (5) offer a more comprehensive description of the psychological effects of MS.

Cognitive Dysfunction

Although once considered symptomatic of only the most severe cases of MS, cognitive dysfunctions have been established as a common symptom of all stages and types of disease (2,11,13). Smith and Schapiro (3) and Polman et al. (9) estimated that as many as 60 to 65 percent of people diagnosed with MS experience some degree of measurable cognitive changes. These changes can affect attention, conceptual reasoning, executive function, and memory. In a recent survey, Roessler et al. (22) found that more than 40 percent of people with MS identified moderate-to-severe cognitive problems. Because MS destroys myelin anywhere in the central nervous system, its associated cognitive impairments cover a wide gamut. The MRI is the best predictor of cognitive status; the greater the number and the more extensive the lesions that can be detected, the more likely the person is to have cognitive impairments as a result of MS (23). Cognitive effects tend to be specific and localized to observable brain lesions; MS does not typically precipitate a decline in general intellectual ability (9).

Affective Disorders

A sizable portion of the overall psychological impact of MS can be viewed in terms of affective disorders that have been shown to accompany the illness. Polman et al. (9) noted that "psychiatric morbidity is increased in MS, with over 50 percent of patients being symptomatic at some stage" (p.85). The most common affective symptoms include irritability, difficulty concentrating, anxiety, bipolar disorder, and depression. Foremost among these is depression. Studies repeatedly show that approximately one-half of all people with MS experience at least one major depressive episode during the course of the illness (24). Clearly, depression is established as a major psychological symptom of MS, but it has yet to be determined whether depressive episodes result from neurological abnormalities or manifest themselves as a psychological response to a serious illness. People with MS are at greater risk for developing depression in all of its forms than are the general population (25). Bipolar disorder is characterized by cyclical patterns of severe depression interspersed with periods of mania and/or euphoria and is diagnosed in approximately 15 percent of people with MS (25). Euphoria, a persistent feeling of well-being and optimism in spite of negative circumstances, is often exhibited by people with MS in isolation of other symptoms (24). Anxiety disorders and other neuroses are also common, although they are often treated effectively with antianxiety medication (24).

Another common psychological symptom of MS is pathological laughing and weeping. A person with MS may break into laughter or begin to weep with slight or no provocation regardless of his or her underlying mood state. Such emotional outbursts can be functionally disabling in and of themselves, making even rudimentary tasks of daily living extremely difficult to perform (25).

Psychological Adjustment

In addition to the cognitive and affective symptoms of MS, the wide-ranging physiological effects of the illness and its capricious course make the process of adjusting to such a debilitating disease a very difficult task. To the extent that MS often renders the individuals more dependent upon others than they were prior to the onset of the illness, friends, family, and coworkers are integral aspects of the adjustment process. A number of factors influence one's overall psychological adjustment to MS. A primary

13

determinant of adjustment is the perceived intrusiveness of the illness—that is, the cumulative effect of (a) functional deficits, physical disabilities, and stressful life events; (b) the unique constellation of signs, symptoms, and treatment constraints associated with an individual's condition; (c) disease activity, life satisfaction, coping style, and knowledge of MS; and (d) personality and social support systems (26). This long list of intrusiveness factors clearly reflects the individual and often unpredictable nature of adjustment to MS.

The far-reaching psychological accompaniments of MS solidify its designation as one of the most difficult diseases to cope with, adjust to, and ultimately accept (15). The nature and progression of physiological and neurological symptoms exact a significant toll on those diagnosed with MS, as well as on their families and friends, and the adjustmental and social issues inherent to MS remain among the most difficult effects of the illness to treat.

Treatment

Just as no certainty exists as to the cause of MS, no treatment modality has been reliably demonstrated to prevent the onset of the illness, progression of central nervous system lesions, or development of new lesions. Moreover, no medical procedure has been developed to alter or dissipate existing lesions. However, adrenocorticotropic hormones and corticosteroids (i.e., prednisone), along with emergent medications such as interferon beta-1a (Avonex and Rebif), interferon beta-1b (Betaseron), glatiramer acetate (Copaxone), mitoxantrone (Novantrone), and natalizumab (Tysabri) (16) have been shown to reduce the severity of exacerbations among some people with MS. Such treatments as fat-free diets, sunflower oil, bee stings, and vitamin supplements have not been proven to be efficacious in definitive clinical trials.

Most MS treatments have been oriented toward catalyzing the body's own immune responses to neurological irregularities. One of the problems in evaluating the efficacy of such treatments is that it is impossible to determine whether improvements or remissions are the results of the treatment or of the natural course of the illness. Physicians have the ability to specify MS treatment regimens to an individual's course and symptoms (2,27), but the search continues for curative treatments that will prevent or arrest the underlying agents of the disease.

Summary

Multiple sclerosis is one of the most prevalent neurological disorders in the United States. Characterized by an unpredictable course, the illness destroys white matter tracts in the central nervous system. Depending on where the nerve damage occurs, people with MS evince a wide range of physiological and psychological symptoms, including fatigue, mobility problems, spasticity, numbness and tingling in the extremities, general weakness, visual impairments, bowel and bladder dysfunction, sexual dysfunction, cognitive disabilities, depression, anxiety, and diminished self-efficacy.

Diagnosing multiple sclerosis has become much easier in recent years with the advent of magnetic resonance imaging and positron emission tomography, but the medical community has been unable as yet to determine the underlying cause of the disease. Most conventional theories concerning the origin of MS espouse an interaction among immunological, viral, and genetic factors as the most likely cause, but attempts to specify that interaction have been inconclusive.

There is presently no cure for MS, but certain recent chemotherapeutic regimens have shown encouraging success in extending the duration of remissions and deintensifying exacerbations of the illness. More research is needed to develop treatments that impede and arrest the progression of this often devastating disease.

Prevalence rates vary widely along gender, cultural, and geographical lines. Women are about twice as likely as men to develop MS, and the illness predominates among individuals of white, Northern European descent. The geographical distribution of MS is also worth noting; two-thirds of the American MS population resides in the northernmost 50 percent of the United States populace.

Multiple sclerosis is distinct from other diseases in etiology, course, range of symptoms, and populational demography. It also has a unique, often deleterious, impact on personal and social functioning. To the extent that a person's work role constitutes an important element of personal and social functioning, the impact of MS on career development is an important consideration for health care providers, rehabilitation professionals, and people with MS and their families. The following chapters provide a comprehensive overview of the work-related issues that people with MS encounter as they cope with this intrusive disease.

References

1. Fraser, R.T., Kraft, G.H., Ehde, D.M., & Johnson, K.L. (2006). *The MS workbook: Living fully with multiple sclerosis.* Oakland, CA: New Harbinger Publications.
2. Schapiro, R.T. (2003). *Managing the Symptoms of Multiple Sclerosis.* 4th Edition. New York: Demos Medical Publishing.

3. Smith, C., & Schapiro, R. (2004). Neurology. In R. Kalb, *Multiple sclerosis: The questions you have the answers you need.* 3rd Edition. New York: Demos Medical Publishing, pp. 7–42.
4. Herndon, R. (2000). Pathology and pathophysiology. In J. Burks & K. Johnson (Eds.), *Multiple sclerosis: Diagnosis, medical management, and rehabilitation.* New York: Demos Medical Publishing, pp. 35–45.
5. Fraser, R., Clemmons, D., & Bennett, F. (2002). *Multiple sclerosis: Psychosocial and vocational interventions.* New York: Demos Medical Publishing.
6. Coyle, P. (2000). Diagnosis and classification of inflammatory demyelinating disorders. In J. Burks & K. Johnson (Eds.). *Multiple sclerosis: Diagnosis, medical management, and rehabilitation.* New York: Demos Medical Publishing, pp. 81–97.
7. Kalb, R. (2007). *Multiple sclerosis: The questions you have the answers you need.* New York: Demos Medical Publishing.
8. Burks, J., & Johnson, K. (2000). *Multiple sclerosis: Diagnosis, medical management, and rehabilitation.* New York: Demos Medical Publishing.
9. Polman, C., Thompson, A., Murray, T., et al. (2006). *Multiple sclerosis: The guide to treatment and management.* New York: Demos Medical Publishing.
10. Barnes, D. (2000). *Multiple sclerosis questions and answers.* Coral Springs, FL: Merit Publishing International.
11. Murray, J. (2000). The history of multiple sclerosis. In J. Burks & K. Johnson (Eds.), *Multiple sclerosis: Diagnosis, medical management, and rehabilitation.* New York: Demos Medical Publishing, pp. 1–32.
12. McAlpine, D., Compston, D., & Lumsden, C. (1955). *Multiple sclerosis.* Edinburgh: E&S Livingstone.
13. Kalb, R. (2004). *Multiple sclerosis: The questions you have the answers you need.* New York: Demos Medical Publishing.
14. Dean, G. (1994). World populations with multiple sclerosis. *Neuroepidemiology, 13,* 1–7.
15. Rumrill, P.D., Jr. (1996). *Employment issues and multiple sclerosis.* New York: Demos Vermande.
16. The National Multiple Sclerosis Society (2006). *The MS Information Source Book,* www.nationalmssociety.org. Retrieved February 18, 2007.
17. Kurtzke, J., & Wallin, M. (2000). Epidemiology. In J. Burks & K. Johnson (Eds.), *Multiple sclerosis: Diagnosis, medical management, and rehabilitation.* New York: Demos Medical Publishing, pp. 49–71.
18. Rumrill, P., & Hennessey, M. (Eds.) (2001). *Multiple sclerosis: A guide for rehabilitation and health care professionals.* Springfield, IL: Charles C Thomas.
19. Poser, C. (1987). Epidemiology and genetics of multiple sclerosis. In L.C. Scheinberg & N.J. Holland (Eds.), *Multiple sclerosis: A guide for patients and their families.* New York: Raven Press, pp. 3–11.
20. Gordon, P., Lewis, M., & Wong, D. (1994). Multiple sclerosis: Strategies for rehabilitation counselors. *Journal of Rehabilitation, 60*(30), 34–38.
21. Foley, F., & Werner, M. (2004). Sexuality. In R. Kalb (Ed.) *Multiple sclerosis: The questions you have the answers you need.* New York: Demos Medical Publishing, pp. 297–328.
22. Roessler, R., Rumrill, P., & Hennessey, M. (2002). *Employment concerns of people with multiple sclerosis: Building a national employment agenda.* Kent, OH: Kent State University Center for Disability Studies, Report Submitted to the National Multiple Sclerosis Society.

23. LaRocca, N., & Sorensen, P. (2004). Cognition. In R. Kalb (Ed.) *Multiple sclerosis: The questions you have the answers you need.* New York: Demos Medical Publishing, pp. 205–232.
24. McReynolds, C., & Koch, L. (2001). Psychological issues. In P. Rumrill & M. Hennessey (Eds.), *Multiple sclerosis: A guide for rehabilitation and health care professionals.* Springfield, IL: Charles C Thomas, pp. 44–78.
25. LaRocca, N. (2004). Stress and emotional issues. In R. Kalb (Ed.), *Multiple sclerosis: The questions you have the answers you need.* New York: Demos Medical Publishing, pp. 273–296.
26. Kalb, R., & Milller, D. (2004). Psychosocial issues. In R. Kalb (Ed.), *Multiple sclerosis: The questions you have the answers you need.* New York,: Demos Medical Publishing, pp. 233–272.
27. Miller, A., Herndon, R., & Bowling, A. (2004). In R. Kalb (Ed.), *Multiple sclerosis: The questions you have the answers you need.* New York: Demos Medical Publishing, pp. 43–80.

Factors Associated with Employment Status

Phillip D. Rumrill, Jr.

Mary L. Hennessey

G IVEN THE WIDE RANGE of medical and psychological symptoms that can accompany multiple sclerosis (MS), the unpredictable disease course and related adjustmental issues, and the negative impact that the illness can have in virtually every aspect of life—as described in Chapter 1—it is not surprising that employment and career development are prominent concerns for people with MS. In this chapter, we describe the most prominent challenges facing people with MS as they attempt to maintain or resume their careers following diagnosis. We begin with a description of the contemporary employment scene for people with MS, and then we discuss known determinants of employment status in an effort to explain the high jobless rate that has plagued the MS community for many years. This chapter sets the stage for subsequent chapters, which detail vocational assessment strategies, employment interventions, federal laws, government programs, and consumer advocacy efforts that can be utilized to assist people with MS in addressing employment-related issues.

Current Employment Scene for People with MS

In contemporary American society, and in most societies across the globe, for that matter, who we are is determined in large measure by what we do for a living (1–3). When we are introduced to strangers at social functions, one of the first points of information we share is our occupation. Psychologically speaking, people often describe their jobs, their employers, and/or their career fields as defining attributes of their identities: "I'm a plumber," "I work at Sears," or "I'm in the restaurant business." Work consumes a considerable portion of a person's sense of self, which stands to reason because experts estimate that American adults spend as much as 70 percent of their waking hours performing tasks related to their jobs (2). This time commitment renders work the single most time-consuming social role for people between the ages of 16 and 65—more time consuming than the roles of parent, spouse or significant other, citizen, friend, and leisurite.

Not only does work occupy our time, it is the primary vehicle through which we earn money, procure goods and services, purchase homes, and save for retirement. Work also provides other, nonmonetary benefits, such as identity formation as mentioned above, socialization, a sense of purpose and accomplishment, group membership (e.g., "I'm in the Teamsters Union"), and access to health care via employer-sponsored insurance (2,4). Sumner (5) connected employment status to life satisfaction and general health, suggesting that people who work are healthier, happier, and more satisfied with their social lives in comparison to people who do not perform paid employment. In a study of Americans with MS, Roessler et al. (6) reported that employed participants had lower levels of perceived stress and higher levels of overall quality of life than did unemployed participants.

From a developmental standpoint, the link between work and identity formation begins early in childhood and continues throughout the life cycle (7,8). As noted in Chapter 1, the onset of MS typically occurs between the ages of 20 and 40—a time that many people regard as the "prime of life." From a career development standpoint, those years are the most active decades of most people's lives. According to Super (8), the period between ages 20 and 40 is marked by (a) exploration (gathering and processing occupational information to formulate career goals), (b) establishment (forging a plan for attainment of those goals and beginning a career), and (c) maintenance (advancing in one's career and attaining his or her goals) activities. For many people with MS, however, the career development process slows and, in many cases, stops after the illness begins to manifest itself.

More than 90 percent of Americans with MS have employment histories; that is, they have worked at some time in the past (9,10). Some

60 percent were still working at the time of diagnosis, even given the lengthy time period that often intervenes between the onset of initial symptoms and confirmed diagnosis (9,11). As the illness progresses, however, people with MS experience a sharp decline in employment; Fraser et al. (12) estimated that only 20 to 30 percent of Americans with MS are employed 15 years after diagnosis, and only 35 to 45 percent of people with MS in the United States are currently employed (10).

Not surprisingly, Americans with MS are gravely concerned about the bleak employment prospects that await them following diagnosis of this intrusive and interruptive disease. In a 2003 survey of 1,310 adults with MS from 10 states and Washington, DC, Roessler et al. (13) found the majority of respondents were dissatisfied with 29 of 32 high-priority employment concerns. Majorities of people with MS were satisfied with only three items: their access to service providers (51 percent), the treatment they received from service providers (61 percent), and the encouragement they received from others to take control of their lives (56 percent). The employment concerns items with the highest dissatisfaction ratings clustered into three thematic categories: implementation and enforcement of the Americans with Disabilities Act, health care and health insurance coverage, and Social Security disability programs. Table 2.1 presents the 29 employment concerns items that were identified as problematic by the majority of respondents, in descending order of dissatisfaction ratings (13, pp. 12–13).

Determinants of Employment Status and Labor Force Participation among People with MS

For many years, medical, psychological, allied health, and rehabilitation researchers have sought to understand why people with MS make a premature, mass exodus from the labor force, usually of their own choosing and often before the disease has rendered them incapable of working. Indeed, among people with MS who are unemployed, 75 percent left their jobs voluntarily (10), 80 percent believe that they retain the ability to work (5), and 75 percent say that they would like to reenter the work force (1). In the endeavor to explain the wholesale disengagement from work that characterizes this well-educated (97 percent of Americans with MS are high school graduates and nearly half hold college degrees [10]), experienced (90 to 95 percent have employment histories, as noted previously) population, the factors associated with employment and unemployment have been a primary focus. The remainder of this chapter

TABLE 2.1: PRIORITY EMPLOYMENT CONCERNS AMONG PEOPLE WITH MS RANKED BY DISSATISFACTION RATINGS

Concern	Percent dissatisfied
People with MS . . .	
have adequate financial help to stay on the job.	81
have access to reasonably priced prescription medications.	78
know their rights regarding job-related physical examinations.	77
have assistance in coping with stress on the job.	76
know about available employment and social services.	75
have their needs considered in the development of Social Security programs.	74
have adequate health insurance so that they can recover and return to work.	73
are treated fairly by employers in the hiring process.	73
receive up-to-date, easily understood information about benefits and work incentives from the Social Security Administration.	72
have opportunities for home-based employment.	72
can work with employers and supervisors who understand the effects of MS.	71
have adequate help in comparing fringe benefits, particularly health insurance coverage, among different job options.	71
have adequate knowledge of the employment protections of Title 1 of the Americans with Disabilities Act.	70
have adequate information about short-and long-term disability.	70
have adequate information on provisions of the Family and Medical Leave Act.	69
can get retraining if it is required to return to work.	68
are considered for other jobs in the same company if their disabilities prevent them from going back to their own jobs.	66
are prepared for real jobs in real work sites.	65
are helped to find employment for which they are prepared.	65
are treated fairly when they apply to work.	64
have transportation needed to travel to and from work.	64
are given support from employers and supervisors after returning to work.	63

(Continued)

TABLE 2.1: CONTINUED

can get help with the cost of assistive devices.	63
are encouraged to work part-time, if full-time is too difficult.	59
receive reasonable accommodations in the workplace.	58
have confidence in their potential to work.	58
can get help in identifying and designing workplace accommodations.	58
receive the same pay as would a non-disabled person.	53
have access to adequate information about Social Security programs.	52

attests to the fact that the medical and psychosocial accompaniments of MS, which at first glance might seem to be the most obvious culprits in the choice to stop working, fail to adequately or sufficiently explain the high rate of unemployment. The symptoms and course of MS have been linked to employment status, but so have a myriad of demographical and environmental variables such as gender, age, socioeconomic status, job type and working conditions, reactions of coworkers and employers, workplace discrimination, and disability benefits. By understanding the factors that are most strongly related to career success on one hand and career attrition on the other for people with MS, readers will more clearly understand the reasons for and targets of the assessment and intervention strategies described in subsequent chapters of this book.

Gender

Although the unemployment rate among Americans with MS is disappointingly low for both sexes, women are significantly less likely to be employed than are men (9,14). LaRocca et al. (15) reported that 80 percent of women with MS were unemployed as compared to 66 percent of men with the illness. Roessler et al. (13) reported similar findings nearly two decades later, revealing jobless rates of 67 percent for women with MS and 51 percent for men with MS in their national survey. Roessler et al. (6) found American women with MS nearly twice as likely to be unemployed as their male counterparts. Canadian citizens with MS appear to experience similar gender disparities when it comes to labor force participation; Edgley et al. (16) reported unemployment rates of 58 and 70 percent for men and women, respectively.

Moreover, other correlates of unemployment seem to affect people with MS differently across gender lines (11). For example, mobility impairment is a strong predictor of job loss for men, whereas women tend to leave the work force before they experience severe physical symptoms (17,18). Also, a lower level of educational attainment has been associated with unemployment for men with MS but not for women (17).

Socioeconomic Status

Both men and women with MS are more likely to leave the work force if they have a spouse who is working (19,18). People with MS who have higher levels of education and/or more money in savings and investments are more likely to be employed than are those in lower socioeconomic strata (16,19,6). This finding may not be surprising given that people with higher levels of education tend to occupy positions that require less physical exertion, and that the physiological effects of MS therefore do not impose work impediments to the same extent as they do for those whose jobs require more physical exertion (20). Rumrill (1) noted that higher-level employees have more flexibility and autonomy in modifying their jobs to meet their MS-related needs. Indeed, employers are generally more likely to accommodate workers who are viewed as talented and essential to the operation of business than they are to meet the needs of less-valued workers (5,21).

Even so, LaRocca (9) suggested that many people with MS who have the financial means to stop working often do so voluntarily, and Duggan et al. (22) reported that three-quarters of unemployed people with MS had left the work force by their own choosing. Unfortunately, those who leave the work force are unlikely to return; LaRocca (9) estimated that only one-third of unemployed Americans with MS have plans to resume their careers in the future.

Age

In a survey of 1,180 Canadians with MS, Edgley et al. (16) found unemployment to increase as a linear function of age. Respondents between the ages of 20 and 29 reported a 38 percent jobless rate, significantly lower than those rates indicated by their counterparts at ages 30 to 39 (57 percent), 40 to 49 (70 percent), 50 to 59 (84 percent), 60 to 69 (87 percent) and 70 and over (93 percent). The relationship between age and unemployment in people with MS has been upheld in several studies in the United States (17,19). LaRocca et al. (15) presented findings indicating a curvilinear direction of that relationship; they found middle-aged people with MS more likely to be employed than either younger or older ones. Rumrill et al. (18) presented similar findings in their employment concerns survey of people with MS in Ohio.

Two factors related to MS and unemployment might help to explain why seasoned, older workers tend to leave the work force before reaching retirement age. First, there is a significant relationship between age and MS-related functional disability (23); as the years pass and the illness progresses, the person becomes less able to meet the physical demands of employment. Second, age is positively associated with socioeconomic status; many older people with MS have the financial means to stop working and do so voluntarily to focus on other pursuits (1).

Physiological Symptoms

Researchers have uncovered a large volume of evidence concerning the impact of the physiological symptoms of MS on employment (see ref. 24). Several studies have revealed the exacerbation and progression of physical symptoms to be strong predictors of job loss. In denoting the most frequently cited reasons that people with MS leave the work force, Rumrill (1) and Fraser et al. (12) noted that as many as 30 percent of unemployed people with MS attribute their jobless status to the physiological effects of the illness, especially fatigue. In a 1985 study, LaRocca et al. (15) found scores on the Kurtzke Disability Status Scale (a measure for determining the severity of physical disability based on neurological examination and functional assessment) to be significant predictors of employment status—the more severe the physical disability, the more likely people with MS were to be unemployed. Gulick et al. (25) found mobility problems to be associated with unemployment in people with MS, as did Kornblith et al. (17) and Rumrill et al. (18). Genevie et al. (19) demonstrated significant relationships between unemployment and such MS symptoms as numbness and tingling, speech problems, visual impairments, pain, fatigue, motor disturbances, and ambulatory problems. Nearly half of unemployed respondents in the survey of people with MS conducted by Edgley et al. (16) cited ambulation difficulties as the primary reason for leaving the work force. Thirty-nine percent described fatigue as the most important contributing factor. On the other hand, Gregory et al. (26) found no relationship between mobility problems and unemployment among people with MS in New Zealand. They suggested that vast improvements in assistive technology over the past several years have mitigated the effects of the physiological symptoms of MS on personal and social functioning. They did cite the inability to work a full day as a common career barrier, but they attributed that difficulty to fatigue and a resultant lack of concentration rather than to mobility problems. Along the same lines, Roessler et al. (6) found no specific physiological symptoms among the most potent predictors of employment status within a random sample of 1,310 Americans with MS. Roessler et al. (6) did find that people with a greater number of MS symptoms, with more persistent symptoms, and with more severe or intrusive symptoms by their own appraisals were more likely to be disengaged from the work force, but physiological symptoms were not singled out as culprits in the mass exodus from the work force that all too often accompanies the onset of this disease.

Course and Disease Progression

In their article on career development and MS, Gordon et al. (27) noted that the most prominent impediment to vocational planning lies in the unpredictable, sometimes progressive, course of the disease. Indeed, numerous characteristics of the disease process have been linked to employment status. Bauer et al.'s (28) now classic study revealed that people with MS with chronic symptom progression were the least likely to be employed, followed, respectively, by people with exacerbating/ progressive symptoms and individuals whose illness was marked by episodic exacerbations and remissions. More recently, Rumrill et al. (18) found people with chronic and progressive MS least likely to be employed. Roessler et al. (6) found that people who experience MS symptoms most or all of the time, especially if the persistent symptoms were greater in number and more severe, are more likely to be unemployed than people with other symptom patterns. More symptoms, more persistent symptoms, and more severe symptoms are generally associated with primary or secondary progressive MS (once known as chronic-progressive MS [29]), so it follows that people with progressive forms of the disease are at greater risk for job loss than people whose MS experience is more episodic and/or less intrusive.

Cognitive Dysfunction

Cognitive deficits associated with MS are, arguably, the most frustrating aspect of the illness (12,30,31). The rate at which one learns new information, skills, and procedures is often diminished (32), as are short-term memory (33), long-term memory (34), and abstract reasoning abilities (35). By their own reports, employees with MS identified significant career maintenance barriers resulting from thought-processing and memory deficits in Roessler and Rumrill's (36) needs assessment study. Rao et al. (37) reported that "cognitively impaired" people with MS were more likely to be unemployed than were "cognitively intact" MS patients. Roessler et al. (6) found people with MS who reported cognitive impairments four times more likely to be unemployed than people with MS who did not report cognitive impairments. Edgley et al. (16) indicated that the frequency of perceived cognitive problems was directly related to the rate of unemployment among people with MS in Canada. Respondents who indicated that they rarely experienced cognitive problems reported an unemployment rate of 53 percent, whereas the unemployment rates for people with MS who described the regularity of cognitive problems as sometimes (67 percent), often (73 percent), and almost always (86 percent) were significantly higher (16).

Psychological and Emotional Factors

The impact of physiological and cognitive impairments on employment status is partially attributable to the location of central nervous system lesions, but the medical effects of the disease fall far short of fully explaining the high rate of work force attrition (38). Many experts believe that the episodic course of MS causes psychological problems which lead to diminished employability. As described in detail in Chapter 1, these problems include depression, anxiety, euphoria, irritability, and emotional instability (30,31).

EMOTIONAL PROBLEMS. Although MS is often accompanied by emotional and/or psychological problems, people with MS are often not fully aware of the extent of these problems and do not generally equate them with job loss (11). LaRocca et al. (15) found that only 2.8 percent of unemployed people with MS considered emotional difficulties to be the primary reason for their job loss. Edgley et al. (16) also noted that self-reported emotional problems had a much smaller impact on employment status than did such factors as gender, age, and physiological symptoms. On the other hand, Genevie et al. (19) found that people with MS who identified problems with emotional lability were significantly less likely to be employed than were those who indicated stable emotional patterns.

JOB SATISFACTION. Job satisfaction has been linked to job tenure and employment status in both the general population (4) and in people with MS (36,39). Roessler and Rumrill (36) found that many people with MS who were employed experienced high levels of dissatisfaction with their jobs. In general, employees with MS were not satisfied with (a) the amount of work that they were expected to do (too much), (b) the amount of pay that they received (too little), (c) their opportunities for advancement (too few), (d) the training that they received on the job (too little), and (e) the recognition afforded them for their work (too little).

JOB MASTERY. Roessler and Rumrill (36) also described job mastery problems as common psychological impediments to career development for people with MS. They reported frequent job mastery concerns among employees with MS in response to such items as (a) considering what I will do in the future, (b) having a plan for where I want to be in my job in the future, and (c) believing that others think I do a good job. These findings suggest that the medical symptoms of MS and the unpredictable disease process make it extremely difficult to formulate and act upon long-term career plans.

SELF-EFFICACY. Rumrill (11,21) proposed the construct of self-efficacy as the "missing link" between MS and unemployment. Self-efficacy comprises two domains of expectancy—efficacy expectations and outcome expectations (40). Efficacy expectations reflect individuals' confidence that they have the skills needed to perform effectively in a given situation. Outcome expectations refer to the likelihood that individuals will actually attempt a certain task, based upon their confidence that task performance would result in desirable outcomes (40).

MS and other severe disabilities often have a negative impact on self-efficacy (41,42). It is also well documented that maintaining a career while coping with a severe disability like MS requires the person to take an active role in overcoming disability-related work limitations (43–45). Thus, the relationship between diminished self-efficacy and unemployment among people with MS can be conceptualized as follows: "They (people with MS) do not believe that they possess the skills required to remove or reduce on-the-job barriers to their productivity (efficacy expectations), nor do they have the confidence that such actions will result in desirable outcomes (outcome expectations)" (44, p. 55).

Workplace Variables
Most contemporary theories of psychology regard human behavior as the product of a complex interaction between personal and environmental

factors (46). A few researchers have examined the work environment for possible explanations for the sharp decline in employment that awaits many people with MS soon after diagnosis.

WORK PERFORMANCE. Gulick et al. (25) viewed the person-environment interaction as an essential consideration in evaluating the work performance of people with MS. Their qualitative study revealed that physical limitations, MS-related symptoms, and environmental factors were interrelated to job performance and, consequently, to job retention. The researchers emphasized the need to empower workers with MS to monitor the progression of their disease and request appropriate job modifications from their employers.

Taking a broad view of work— one including employment, activities of daily living, and coping with MS symptoms—Gulick (47) attributed diminished work performance to work impediments such as mobility problems, fine motor difficulties, deterioration of general body state, cognitive dysfunction, pain, and environmental barriers. She suggested that people with MS could improve their work performance via such work enhancers as job adjustments, environmental adjustments and assistive technology, social support, and healthful self-care practices.

CAREER ADJUSTMENT BARRIERS: WORKSITE ACCESSIBILITY AND PERFORMANCE OF ESSENTIAL FUNCTIONS. The Minnesota Theory of Work Adjustment (4) holds that job tenure (i.e., how long a worker keeps his or her job) is a function of satisfaction and satisfactoriness. Satisfaction refers to the extent to which a job provides sufficient internal and external reinforcement for the individual, whereas satisfactoriness reflects how well the person performs the job. Crites (48) proposed job tenure (i.e., satisfaction + satisfactoriness) to be largely determined by one's ability to overcome thwarting conditions, or barriers, at work.

Conceptualizing the medical and psychological effects of MS as internal barriers to career adjustment, Roessler and Rumrill (36) examined perceived worksite barriers for their relationship to feelings of job satisfaction and job mastery (i.e., satisfactoriness) among a sample of employees with MS in Indiana and Kentucky. Using the Work Experience Survey (WES) (49), the researchers found that the number of disability-related barriers to (a) worksite accessibility and (b) performance of essential job functions correlated significantly and positively with the number of satisfaction and mastery problems reported by respondents. As a result, Rumrill (11) developed a simple prediction equation to assess a worker's risk of job loss: "The more accessibility and essential function barriers one perceives on the job, the lower the levels of job satisfaction and mastery and, thus, the greater the risk of job loss" (p. 39).

EMPLOYER ATTITUDES AND REACTIONS OF COWORKERS. Another worksite factor that bears on people's ability to retain employment while coping with MS is the reaction of their employers and coworkers. This is not to imply, however, that employer attitudes toward people with MS are always negative. Sumner (5) reported that many employers have gone to great lengths to educate themselves about MS and to accommodate workers who are coping with the disease. He identified open communication and a willingness on the part of employee and employer to understand one another's concerns as the key ingredients to successful job retention for people with MS.

Ketelaer et al. (50) found that employer attitudes and interactions with coworkers influenced employees' willingness to request MS-related accommodations at work. Rumrill et al. (51) connected the act of requesting on-the-job accommodations to self-efficacy, which has been associated with MS and employment status in several investigations (21,36,41,43). Putting these findings together forges a direct link between environmental and personal factors related to the employment of people with MS: reactions of employers and coworkers influence the employee's willingness to ask for needed help on the job; willingness to ask for help influences self-efficacy, and vice versa; the reciprocal relationship between self-efficacy and willingness to ask for help influences the person's prospects for continued employment (11).

JOB TYPE AND WORKING CONDITIONS. In their 1985 study, LaRocca et al. (15) asserted that, although occupational type was related to a person's overall psychosocial adjustment to MS, it was unrelated to employment status. Such factors as disability level, age, gender, and educational attainment were much stronger predictors of job retention and loss within the American MS population. More recently, however, Ketelaer et al. (50) reported that people employed in the medical field and in jobs that required them to work out-of-doors, stand for long periods of time, and/or exert physical strength were far more likely to lose their jobs than were those working under other occupational conditions. Rumrill et al. (52) found that well-educated, professional-level workers with MS had fewer employment problems and, consequently, more optimism about continued career success than did workers in other job categories.

30

Duggan et al. (22) simply asked unemployed people with MS why they had left their jobs. Approximately 75 percent reported stopping work voluntarily, but worksite barriers were frequently cited as reasons for that choice. These on-the-job obstacles included less-than-helpful employee assistance programs and a lack of reasonable accommodations. Many respondents believed that they could have benefited from such assistance as home-based work, education for their employers about MS, and individual employment counseling. A number of respondents also felt that information concerning the Americans with Disabilities Act, legal rights, health insurance, and Social Security Disability Insurance would have helped them to retain employment. It is important to note that people with MS seldom attribute their all-too-frequent unemployment to issues of absenteeism, safety, or interpersonal conflicts with coworkers and supervisors (11,22). It should also be pointed out that people with MS often leave the work force for non-MS–related reasons. LaRocca et al. (15) revealed that 37 percent of unemployed people with MS had left their jobs due to pregnancy, marriage, relocation, or retirement.

Workplace Discrimination

Technically speaking, the choice to leave the work force is most often made by individuals with MS themselves, but it is not known to what extent the phenomenon of discrimination in the workplace "helps" people with MS to make that choice. What is known is that perceived discrimination is a major obstacle to continued employment following diagnosis with MS, and that people with MS often believe that their employers treat them unfairly in comparison to nondisabled workers. Indeed, Rumrill and Hennessey (24) described workplace discrimination as the unifying feature of the employment experience for Americans with MS, suggesting that it is the number one explanation for the high rate of workforce attrition that follows the onset of the illness.

That assertion is borne in empirical research findings. In the national survey conducted by Roessler et al. (10), no fewer than six items related to implementation of the Americans with Disabilities Act (ADA) and the Family and Medical Leave Act (FMLA) were reported among the 12 most prominent employment-related problems identified by Americans with MS. Specifically, the majority of respondents reported having been treated unfairly in the hiring process by employers (73 percent), having been denied reasonable accommodations (58 percent), having received lower pay than their nondisabled peers (53 percent), being refused schedule modifications that would have enabled them to continue working (59 percent), having received inadequate health insurance coverage (73 percent), and having received little or no information about their legal rights from employers (69 percent).

Between 1992 and 2003, the United States Equal Employment Opportunity Commission received and resolved 3,669 allegations of employment discrimination from people with MS under Title I of the ADA. Allegations of unlawful termination constituted the most commonly cited form of workplace discrimination (29.9 percent), followed in descending order by complaints related to reasonable accommodations (21.9 percent), terms and conditions of employment (9.8 percent), harassment (6.7 percent), hiring (3.8 percent), discipline (3.4 percent), constructive discharge (i.e., creating a work environment that makes it impossible for the person to continue working; 3.0 percent), layoff (2.8 percent), and promotion (2.5 percent). People with MS filing ADA Title I allegations were mostly female (66.5 percent), predominantly white (76.1 percent), and of mid-career age on average (M = 42.47 years, SD = 8.54). Allegations were most often filed against employers in the South United States Census tracking region (35.7 percent), and employers in the service, financial, insurance, and real estate industries were most often the subjects of ADA Title I complaints.

In comparison to ADA Title I complainants with other disabilities, people with MS were more likely than people with other disabilities to allege discrimination under Title I of the ADA in the areas of reasonable accommodations, terms and conditions of employment, constructive discharge, and demotion; less likely to allege discrimination in the area of hiring; and more likely to have their allegations of discrimination resolved in their favor by the United States Equal Employment Opportunity Commission (EEOC) (53–55). Even though people with MS do prevail in ADA Title I complaints to the EEOC at a higher rate than people with other disabilities, the troubling fact remains that 75 percent of all ADA Title I allegations filed by people with MS since 1992 have been found to have insufficient merit as to warrant a claim of discrimination.

The problem of workplace discrimination was further underscored in several focus groups of people with MS conducted by Roessler et al. (13). Focus group members identified discrimination and unfair treatment at work as one of the top agenda items for improving the rate of labor force participation among people with MS. Similarly, 38 percent of callers into

Kent State University's MS Employment Assistance Service hotline since 1999 have sought assistance with interpreting their legal rights and/or redressing employer discrimination (1).

Disability Benefits

It is well-documented that people with MS who receive disability benefits from private insurers or from government agencies face extreme difficulties in restarting their careers. Indeed, the benefits paid by most long-term disability insurance carriers and the Social Security Administration's two disability programs (i.e., Social Security Disability Insurance [SSDI] and Supplemental Security Income [SSI]) are predicated on the beneficiary being too disabled to work (56). This requirement provides a powerful systemic disincentive that keeps thousands of Americans with MS from participating in the labor force. Once they have been adjudicated as too severely disabled to work by either long-term disability insurers or Social Security (or sometimes both), they integrate the external confirmation of their disabled status into their own self-concepts—self-concepts that do not include the role of worker (57). From that point on in the vast majority of cases, unemployment and receipt of disability benefits conjoin in a self-fulfilling prophecy for people with MS (24). According to Fraser et al. (58), people with MS progress from active employment to short-term disability insurance, long-term disability insurance, and, finally, SSDI at higher and faster rates than people with most other disabilities. Once on SSDI, the "too disabled to work" message has already registered loud and clear, and over time it would seem to become impervious to alternative messages of employability. According to Fraser et al., (12) less than 1 percent of Americans with MS who receive SSDI benefits will ever resume gainful employment.

Lest readers conclude that archival data from insurance carriers and the Social Security Administration are the only bases for our assertion that disability benefits negatively impact employment, focus groups of people with MS identified work disincentives in SSDI, SSI, and long-term disability insurance among their three most important reasons for the low employment rate among adults with MS. Also in the voices of people with MS, no fewer than 52 percent of the 2,411 people with MS who participated in Kent State University's nationwide MS Employment Assistance Service between 2001 and 2006 had concerns related to long-term disability insurance or Social Security programs (1).

Summary

Existing research has identified a number of factors that are associated with the career development difficulties faced by people with MS. Demographical characteristics such as gender, socioeconomic status, and age are related to unemployment in people with MS. Specifically, women, older workers, and those with lower levels of education are most likely to be unemployed. As might be expected, the physiological symptoms of MS also explain some of the variance in employment status. Physical limitations (especially mobility problems) and fatigue are commonly cited reasons for job loss. To a lesser extent, visual impairments, loss of coordination, and incontinence have also been attributed. In addition, disease-related variables such as age at onset, duration of illness, number and persistence of symptoms, and the progression of symptoms have been shown to predict whether one continues working while coping with MS.

Cognitive and other psychological problems have a significant impact on employment. Memory problems, thought-processing difficulties, emotional instability, job satisfaction and mastery concerns, and low self-efficacy have all been linked to poor prospects for job retention. At the workplace itself, many on-the-job variables have been examined for their contributions to the career maintenance difficulties experienced by people with MS. These include the performance of essential functions, worksite accessibility, employer attitudes and coworker reactions, and the availability of reasonable accommodations. Workplace discrimination, long viewed as the ultimate behavioral manifestation of negative attitudes toward workers with MS, continues to be a pervasive impediment to the job retention and career maintenance efforts of Americans with MS. Last but not least are work disincentives in the Social Security Administration's programs and in long-term disability insurance policies, most of which are predicated on the person being too disabled to work.

Taken in aggregate, research examining the determinants of employment status and labor force participation among people with MS have provided considerable insight into the issues that confront this experienced, well-trained, and yet all-too-often disenfranchised group of workers as they attempt to maintain their careers while dealing with a highly intrusive chronic illness. Chapter 3 and 4 highlight assessment and intervention strategies that medical and rehabilitation professionals have used to combat the devastating toll that MS can exact on one's career development.

If Chapter 2 indicates how far we still have to go in righting the career ladder for people with MS, Chapters 3 and 4 provide some directions and strategies regarding how to get there.

References

1. Rumrill, P. (2006). Help to stay at work: Vocational rehabilitation strategies for people with multiple sclerosis. *Multiple Sclerosis in Focus, 7*, 14–18.
2. Wehman, P. (2006). *Life beyond the classroom: Transition strategies for young people with disabilities*. Baltimore: Paul H. Brookes.
3. Zunker, V.G. (1994). *Foundations of career counseling: Applied concepts of life planning.* Pacific Grove, CA: Brooks/Cole Publishing.
4. Dawis, R., & Lofquist, L. (1984). *A psychological theory of work adjustment.* Minneapolis: University of Minnesota Press.
5. Sumner, G. (1997). *Project Alliance: A job retention program for employees with chronic illnesses and their employers*. New York: National Multiple Sclerosis Society.
6. Roessler, R., Rumrill, P., & Fitzgerald, S. (2004). Predictors of employment status for people with multiple sclerosis. *Rehabilitation Counseling Bulletin, 47*(2), 97–103.
7. Hennessey, M. (2004). An examination of the employment and career development concerns of postsecondary students with disabilities: Results of a tri-regional survey. Doctoral Dissertation. Kent, OH: Kent State University.
8. Super, D. (1980). A life-span, life-space approach to career development. *Journal of Vocational Behavior, 16*, 282–298.
9. LaRocca, N.G. (1995). *Employment and multiple sclerosis*. New York: National Multiple Sclerosis Society.
10. Roessler, R., Rumrill, P., & Hennessey, M. (2002). *Employment concerns of people with multiple sclerosis: Building a national employment agenda*. Kent, OH: Kent State University Center for Disability Studies, Report Submitted to the National Multiple Sclerosis Society.
11. Rumrill, P.D., Jr. (1996). *Employment issues and multiple sclerosis*. New York: Demos Vermande.
12. Fraser, R., Clemmons, D., & Bennett, F. (2002). *Multiple sclerosis: Psychosocial and vocational interventions*. New York: Demos Medical Publishing.
13. Roessler, R., Rumrill, P., Hennessey, M., et al. (2003). Perceived strengths and weaknesses in employment policies and practices among people with multiple sclerosis: Results of a national survey. *Work: A Journal of Prevention, Assessment, and Rehabilitation, 21*(1), 25–36.
14. Roessler, R., Fitzgerald, S., Rumrill, P., & Koch, L. (2001). Determinants of employment status among people with multiple sclerosis. *Rehabilitation Counseling Bulletin, 45*(1), 31–39.
15. LaRocca, N.G., Kalb, R., Scheinberg, L.C., & Kendall, P. (1985). Factors associated with unemployment of patients with multiple sclerosis. *Journal of Chronic Diseases, 38*, 203–210.
16. Edgley, K., Sullivan, M., & Dehoux, E. (1991). A survey of multiple sclerosis, part 2: Determinants of employment status. *Canadian Journal of Rehabilitation, 4*(3), 127–132.
17. Kornblith, A.B., LaRocca, N.G., & Baum, H.M. (1986). Employment in individuals with multiple sclerosis. *International Journal of Rehabilitation Research, 9*, 155–165.

18. Rumrill, P., (1999). Effects of a social competence training program on accommodation request activity, situational self-efficacy, and Americans with Disabilities Act knowledge among employed people with visual impairments and blindness. *Journal of Vocational Rehabilitation, 12*(1), 25–31.

19. Genevie, L., Kallos, J., & Struenig, E. (1987). Job retention among people with multiple sclerosis. *Journal of Neurological Rehabilitation, 1,* 131–135.

20. Rumrill, P., Koch, L., & Reed, C. (1998). Career maintenance and multiple sclerosis. *Journal of Job Placement and Development, 14*(1), 11–17.

21. Rumrill, P. (1993). Increasing the frequency of accommodation requests among employed people with multiple sclerosis. Unpublished Doctoral Dissertation. Fayetteville: University of Arkansas.

22. Duggan, E., Fagan, P., & Yateman, S. (1993). *Employment factors among individuals with multiple sclerosis.* Unpublished manuscript. New York: National Multiple Sclerosis Society.

23. Wineman, N.M. (1990). Adaptation to multiple sclerosis: The role of social support, functional disability, and perceived uncertainty. *Nursing Research, 39,* 294–299.

24. Rumrill, P., & Hennessey, M. (Eds.) (2001). *Multiple sclerosis: A guide for rehabilitation and health care professionals.* Springfield, IL: Charles C Thomas.

25. Gulick, E.E., Yam, M., & Touw, M.M. (1989). Work performance by persons with multiple sclerosis: Conditions that impede or enable the performance of work. *International Journal of Nursing Studies, 26*(4), 301–311.

26. Gregory, R., Disler, P., & Firth, S. (1993). Employment and multiple sclerosis in New Zealand. *Journal of Occupational Rehabilitation, 3*(2), 113–117.

27 .Gordon, P.A., Lewis, M.D., & Wong, D. (1994). Multiple sclerosis: Strategies for rehabilitation counselors. *Journal of Rehabilitation, 60*(3), 34–38.

28. Bauer, H., Firnhaber, W., & Winkler, W. (1965). Prognostic criteria in multiple sclerosis. *Annals of the New York Academy of Sciences, 122,* 542–551.

29. Schapiro, R. (2003). *Managing the symptoms of multiple sclerosis.* New York, NY: Demos Medical Publishing.

30. Kalb, R. (2007). *Multiple sclerosis: The questions you have the answers you need.* New York: Demos Medical Publishing.

31. McReynolds, C., & Koch, L. (2001). Psychological issues. In P. Rumrill and M. Hennessey (Eds.), *Multiple sclerosis: A guide for rehabilitation and health care professionals.* Springfield, IL: Charles C Thomas, pp. 44–78.

32. Franklin, G., Nelson, L., Filley, C., & Heaton, R. (1989). Cognitive loss in multiple sclerosis: Case reports and review of the literature. *Archives of Neurology, 46*(2), 162–167.

33. Grant, I., McDonald, W.I., Trimble, M., et al. (1984). Deficient learning and memory in early and middle phases of multiple sclerosis. Journal of Neurology, Neurosurgery, and Psychiatry, *47,* 250–255.

34. Rao, S., Leo, G., & St. Aubin-Faubert, P. (1989). A critical review of the Luria-Nebraska neuropsychological literature. *International Journal of Clinical Neuropsychology, 11*(3), 137–142.

35. Halligan, F.R., Reznikoff, M., Friedman, H., & LaRocca, N.G. (1988). Cognitive dysfunction and change in multiple sclerosis. *Journal of Clinical Psychology, 44*(4), 540–548.

36. Roessler, R., & Rumrill, P. (1995). The relationship of perceived worksite barriers to job mastery and job satisfaction for employed people with multiple sclerosis. *Rehabilitation Counseling Bulletin, 39*(1), 2–14.

37. Rao, S., Leo, G., Ellington, L., et al. (1991). Cognitive dysfunction in multiple sclerosis: Impact on employment and social functioning. *Neurology, 41*(5), 692–696.

38. LaRocca, N.G., & Hall, H.L. (1990). Multiple sclerosis program: A model for neuropsychiatric disorders. *New Directions for Mental Health Services, 45*, 49–64.

39. Roessler, R., & Rumrill, P. (1998). Reducing worksite barriers to enhance job satisfaction: An important post-employment service for employees with chronic illnesses. *Journal of Vocational Rehabilitation, 10*(3), 219–229.

40. Bandura, A. (1986). *Social foundations of thought and action: A social cognitive theory.* Englewood Cliffs, NJ: Prentice-Hall.

41. Devins, G.M., & Seland, T.P. (1987). Emotional impact of multiple sclerosis: Recent findings and suggestions for future research. *Psychological Bulletin, 101*, 363–375.

42. Strauser, D. (1995). Applications of self-efficacy theory to rehabilitation counseling. *Journal of Rehabilitation, 61*(7), 17–22.

43. Gecas, V. (1989). The social psychology of self-efficacy. *Annual Review of Sociology, 15*, 291–316.

44. Roessler, R., & Rumrill, P.D., Jr. (1994). Strategies for enhancing career maintenance self-efficacy of people with multiple sclerosis. *Journal of Rehabilitation, 60*(4), 54–59.

45. Rumrill, P. (1999). Effects of a social competence training program on accommodation request activity, situational self-efficacy, and Americans with Disabilities Act knowledge among employed people with visual impairments and blindness. *Journal of Vocational Rehabilitation, 12*(1), 25–31.

46. Kosciulek, J. (1993). Advances in trait-and-factor theory: A person x environment approach to rehabilitation counseling. *Journal of Applied Rehabilitation Counseling, 24*(2), 11–14.

47. Gulick, E.E. (1992). Model for predicting work performance among persons with multiple sclerosis. *Nursing Research, 41*(5), 266–272.

48. Crites, J. (1976). A comprehensive model of career development in early adulthood. *Journal of Vocational Behavior, 9*, 105–118.

49. Roessler, R. (1995). *The Work Experience Survey.* Fayetteville, AR: Arkansas Research and Training Center in Vocational Rehabilitation.

50. Ketelaer, P., Crijns, H., Gausin, J., & Bouwen, R. (1993). *Multiple sclerosis and employment: Synthesis report.* Brussels: Belgian Ministry of Labour and Employment.

51. Rumrill, P.D., Jr., Roessler, R.T., & Denny, G.S. (1997). Increasing participation in the accommodation request process among employed people with multiple sclerosis: A career maintenance self-efficacy intervention. *Journal of Job Placement, 13*(1), 5–9.

52. Rumrill, P., Roessler, R., & Koch, L. (1999). Surveying the employment concerns of people with multiple sclerosis: A participatory action research approach. *Journal of Vocational Rehabilitation, 12*(2), 75–82.

53. Rumrill, P., Roessler, R., McMahon, B., & Fitzgerald, S. (2005). Multiple sclerosis and workplace discrimination: The national Equal Employment Opportunity Commission Americans with Disabilities Act research project. *Journal of Vocational Rehabilitation, 23*(3), 179–188.

54. Rumrill, P., Roessler, R., Unger, D., & Vierstra, C. (2004). Title I of the Americans with Disabilities Act and Equal Employment Opportunity Commission case resolution patterns involving people with multiple sclerosis. *Journal of Vocational Rehabilitation, 20*(3), 171–176.

55. Unger, D., Rumrill, P., Roessler, R., & Stacklin, R. (2004). A comparative analysis of employment discrimination complaints filed by people with multiple sclerosis

and individuals with other disabilities. *Journal of Vocational Rehabilitation, 20*(3), 165–170.

56. Marini, I. (2003). What rehabilitation counselors should know to assist Social Security beneficiaries in becoming employed. *Work: A Journal of Prevention, Assessment, and Rehabilitation, 21*(1), 37–44.

57. Roessler, R., & Rumrill, P. (2003). Multiple sclerosis and employment barriers: A systemic approach. *Work: A Journal of Prevention, Assessment, and Rehabilitation, 21*(1), 17–23.

58. Fraser, R., McMahon, B., & Dancyzk-Hawley, C. (2004). Progression of disability benefits: A perspective on multiple sclerosis. *Journal of Vocational Rehabilitation, 19*(3), 173–179.

3 Vocational Assessment Strategies*

Richard T. Roessler

O NE THEME RECURS THROUGHOUT this book: multiple sclerosis (MS) is a severe mid-career disability that presents significant challenges to adults who are determined to resume or retain employment. Indicative of the complications associated with the disease, the unemployment rate for people with MS equals or exceeds that reported by the general population of adults with disabilities (1–4). For the most part, barriers to the retention of employment result from the gravity, pervasiveness, and unpredictability of the symptoms themselves (5). At the same time, these symptoms tend to have a cumulative psychological effect that results in feelings of both uncertainty and powerlessness regarding one's life and future (6). Feelings of uncertainty about one's future status, in turn, serve to magnify the impact of individual physical and cognitive symptoms associated with the disease process (7). This chapter describes assessment strategies that help to clarify the way that MS both impairs functioning in career roles and

---

* This chapter addresses strategies for assessing the medical, psychological, and social aspects of career development for people with MS. It is intended primarily for health care professionals, social workers, psychologists, and rehabilitation practitioners who have a basic working knowledge of psychometric principles. For the benefit of readers who do not have a background in measurement, technical terms are defined in the text.

produces feelings of uncertainty and powerlessness about the future. As Power and Hershenson (8) stressed, the probability that a person will return to work depends in large part on the impact of disability on work competencies and life outlook in terms of work goals and motivation.

Assessments recommended for people with MS provide insights into the personal preferences, functional limitations, rehabilitation outlook, and perceived barriers that affect success in coping with the effects of physical and psychological symptoms of the illness. The reader is reminded, however, of one of the basic premises of psychological assessment supported by Goldberg's research (9): in the case of people with adventitious disabilities such as MS, the best predictors of future interests, values, and vocational accomplishments are the person's past interests, values, and vocational accomplishments. Indeed, for acquired disabling conditions, prior commitments and preferences have more influence on the person's vocational choice than does the severity of the disability (9). Hence, rehabilitation professionals should concentrate first on helping individuals with MS maintain continuity in their vocational lives by retaining employment held before the onset of disability, turning to other vocational assessments and placement strategies when necessary to identify transferable skills and potential jobs with compatible skill demands.

A Philosophy of Assessment

Because of their impact on individual functioning in a variety of areas (mobility, strength, cognition, and vision), the symptoms of MS are disruptive to the person's career in the broadest sense of the term *career*. For example, the more encompassing career development theories define career as including multiple life roles such as employee, citizen, learner, family member, and participant in leisure activities (10). Hence, although this chapter focuses on issues of vocational evaluation, it does not intend to imply that the effect of MS on the other daily living and community roles is unimportant. The interdependence of career roles is stressed, requiring that the rehabilitation professional explore how MS affects multiple career roles and life functions (11,12) and how limitations in performance of these roles and functions impinge on the person's capability to seek, acquire, and retain employment.

In addition to the career emphasis, the philosophy of assessment underlying this chapter includes a person-in-environment perspective that integrates the traditional trait and factor approach with the ecological approach. The trait and factor paradigm is retained because it defines personal variables that are fairly stable even in the face of a significant disability such as MS. Such attributes of the person as vocational interests, aptitudes, skills, self-concept, and preferences for work climates and reinforcers fall into the trait/factor category (13–15).

The ecological perspective is also useful because it stresses that environmental variables are equally important for understanding the vocational outcomes of a person with a disability. As Dobren (16) noted, these ecological variables include the attitudes of others (e.g., reactions of family and employer to the disability and resumption of employment) and the presses in the environment (e.g., nature of the tasks or expectations that define the career setting in which the person is expected to function). Dobren (16) also described how severe disabilities such as MS alter the context in which the person functions by creating new variables with which the person has little or no experience, such as architectural barriers, attitudes of physicians and other health care providers, and financial disincentives posed by disability benefit programs. Therefore, the assessor must have a perspective that encompasses the person, the context, and the interaction of the two. One must understand the tasks and expectations of the job the person holds (environment) to know which disability-related limitations (person) create significant barriers to performance of essential job functions. Because the effects of MS vary so widely among individuals, on-the-job barriers must be considered on the basis of each person's specific job duties. For example, a high school mathematics teacher coping with mobility restrictions as a result of MS is less vocationally handicapped than a farmer or construction worker dealing with the same or even less severe mobility impairments.

As noted, focusing assessment on physical limitations alone without examining the demands of a specific career role can provide only a partial understanding of the person's needs. Knowledge of both allows the professional to intervene with both the individual's capacities and the demands of the environment. Thus, coupling the trait and factor perspective with the ecological outlook provides a more encompassing view of assessment and its implications. With the dual (person/environment) point of view, the professional understands that interventions are not directed solely at changing the person. They also must affect the situation in which the person functions, with the end result being congruence between the job demands and the person's capabilities as mediated by the accommodative strategies that include job restructuring,

41

technology utilization, and flexible scheduling (17). The remainder of this chapter provides an overview of assessment strategies and measurements that, when viewed in their entirety, are sensitive to the person's characteristics (i.e., strengths and limitations) and the demands of the setting. Results from such instruments provide practical information on the person's needs for skill-building and self-exploration experiences, technology utilization, and environmental modifications.

Capitalizing on Continuity

Given the research-based conclusion that the best predictors of future vocational preferences are past vocational preferences (9), the rehabilitation professional working with people with MS should first involve the person in examining the feasibility of returning to the same job with the same employer as quickly as possible (18). If such employment is possible, the next step involves identifying barriers at the workplace that impede vocational success and the reasonable accommodations that will reduce or remove those barriers. An assessment strategy for identifying workplace barriers, the Work Experience Survey (WES) (19), is described later in this chapter.

If adults with MS cannot return to their same jobs/same employers, rehabilitation professionals can assist them in completing a vocational analysis, with the end goal being identification of similar or related employment roles available in the local community. Described in recent rehabilitation resources (17), the vocational analysis may be no more involved than reviewing intake interview information and existing occupational information resources. For example, Power (20) provided a vocationally oriented intake interview schedule that guides individuals through a discussion of their interests as revealed in past work, hobbies, and leisure activities; educational achievements and preferences; preferred work demands and conditions; aptitudes; and nature and quality of social support network. This personal information directs the person with MS and the counselor in their efforts to use vocational information resources to identify and explore feasible vocational alternatives.

Many helpful sources of occupational information are available from the United States Department of Labor such as the O*NET (21), the *Guide for Occupational Exploration* (22), and the annual *Occupational Outlook Handbook* (23,24). Information in these published and web-based resources will help individuals and the rehabilitation professionals assisting them in the process of identifying feasible job options and developing job-seeking plans.

The O*NET website is useful because it enables a person to complete a vocational self-evaluation that results in a skill profile that can be related to task demands of a wide variety of jobs. Results from the O*NET website search includes a listing of the jobs matching the person's skill profile, allowing the person to access comprehensive job descriptions of positions of interest. The individual may also enter the title of a job previously held in the O*NET and review job descriptions of related jobs. In addition, the O*NET has relevant links to other informative websites such as the Job Accommodation Network (JAN), which provides a wealth of information on disabilities, functional limitations, and reasonable accommodations. The JAN accommodation resource also lists vendors for products that the person may wish to research and, possibly, purchase as a part of a job maintenance or return-to-work plan. For workers with MS, useful accommodations listed in the JAN website address such concerns as visual limitations, memory loss, and fatigue.

For current information on jobs of interest located through the O*NET search, the *Occupational Outlook Handbook*, published by the U.S. Department of Labor, is a useful resource (25). Current information is provided on the educational and training requirements for the position, the occupational outlook for the job, and the salary/wage range typically associated with the position. Divided into occupational categories, the Handbook lists both primary and related occupational roles in those categories to encourage individuals to think broadly about their vocational possibilities.

The *Guide for Occupational Exploration* (GOE) (22) provides yet another strategy for capitalizing on continuity. Using the GOE, the individual with MS and the rehabilitation professional can identify one of the 14 interest areas in which the person's prior job fell (e.g., artistic, business detail, sales and marketing). If individuals can no longer perform a particular job, then they can scan other job titles in that interest category to identify feasible vocational roles. Individuals may also do vocational exploration using the GOE by identifying job titles in interest categories containing work activities that appeal to them. Should they need more information on any of these jobs, they may return to the O*NET to study the skill profile of the job or to the *Enhanced Occupational Outlook* (24) to review educational requirements and employment projections.

Based on information on the physical demands and job duties of positions in resources such as the O*NET, the Handbook, and the

GOE, the rehabilitation professional can help the individual with MS evaluate the feasibility of vocational alternatives in terms of job/person match or congruence (26,27). Parker et al. (27) listed the person and job variables that must be considered in establishing this person/job match. For example, using intake interview information and existing evaluation data, the rehabilitation professional can create a synthesis of the person's medical and educational history, past vocational training, work history and preferred work activities, current financial situation, and current work-related strengths and limitations (17). This case history is extremely important because research with people who have MS indicates that elements of a person's history are related to employment outcomes. Poor employment outcomes are associated with (a) the chronic progression of MS; (b) greater physical involvement including spasticity, lack of coordination, and disturbances in bowel and bladder function; and (c) being female and older (3,4,28). Larsen (29) reported that adjustment scores in the vocational domain for people with MS were higher for those who had employment histories or had attended college.

As a result of the vocational analysis, the person has a list of feasible vocational alternatives that should be evaluated for (a) compatibility with his or her skills and interests and (b) availability in the local community. Recommending a job analysis to estimate person/job compatibility, Patterson (30) stressed the need for specific information about work methods and techniques, work output or products, desired characteristics of workers, and the context of the work. The size and stability of the company, availability of employer-provided transportation for employees, and the employer's history of support for and retention of people with disabilities are examples of other types of valuable information about the employer (27).

The most promising job titles identified in the vocational analysis provide the foundation for beginning a traditional job search strategy including such steps as building one's job lead network, accessing information on current job openings, organizing the job search, and recoding the results of job-seeking contacts. LaRocca and Hall (31) described the use of job-seeking groups in their MS Job-Raising program (see Chapter 4), which included didactic instruction in job-seeking and networking as well as personal support among people with MS.

Other strategies exist for initiating the vocational analysis process that capitalize on continuity; that is, the desirability of helping the person with MS resume employment similar to that held before the onset or exacerbation of symptoms. One technique requires knowledge of the work reinforcers (those factors that encourage a person to continue working) available in a job and the titles of other jobs providing similar types of reinforcers. In the Minnesota Theory of Work Adjustment (26), 20 discrete work reinforcers are defined, such as creativity, compensation, authority, and activity. Each job has a characteristic pattern of reinforcers, and each person has a characteristic set of preferences for these reinforcers. To increase the probability of job satisfaction, people with MS must identify new job titles that both are available in the local community and provide access to preferred reinforcers, while still involving them in job duties compatible with their existing skills and physical capacities.

Although estimates of reinforcer preferences on the part of the person and reinforcer availability on the part of the job may be generated from interviews with the person and his or her supervisors and coworkers, a written assessment measure that the person with MS can complete is also available. The Minnesota Importance Questionnaire (MIQ) enables respondents to indicate their personal preferences among the 20 work reinforcers. The resulting needs profile of the person is related to information on the work reinforcers characteristic of a wide range of jobs, and a list of job/person matches is produced as an outcome of the computer scoring process for the MIQ. This list of job titles includes positions that the person would find satisfying based on the need/reinforcer match principle (26,32,33). The next steps are to identify compatible positions available in the local community and to assist the person in organizing a job search plan targeted at those jobs and employers.

Research with the Minnesota Theory of Work Adjustment (33) demonstrated that satisfaction with one's work is only one of the factors that affect tenure on the job. The other important factor is satisfactoriness on the job; that is, the ability to perform the job as evaluated by one's supervisor or employer. Consistent with the ecological perspective advocated earlier, satisfactoriness is a function of the person's being able to perform job-specific tasks in a manner that meets the employer's quantity and quality standards. Although the potential for job satisfactoriness should be analyzed in detail prior to placement, it is also possible to assess on-the-job satisfactoriness using the Minnesota Satisfactoriness Scales (MSS) (26,32,33) as a postemployment service. Completed by the supervisor or employer, the MSS contains items addressing the person's work capacities, comparability with other workers in the position, and suitability for a pay raise and promotion. If gathered early enough in the worker's adjustment to the new position, MSS data can highlight areas in which the person needs additional support, training, or accommodations to cope more effectively with the demands of the new position. If made as soon as possible, such postplacement adjustments increase the probability of satisfactoriness, which, when coupled with satisfaction, is predictive of long-term tenure on the job.

Career Role Performance

In keeping with the career theme and ecological perspective described earlier, Gulick (34,35) presented several assessments useful with people who have MS. Defining work as activity that requires the expenditure of energy to maintain the person's existence, self-esteem, or remuneration, she developed the Work Assessment Scale (WAS), which enables people with MS to describe the factors that impede the capacity to do work (WAS-I) and the factors that have potential to reduce or remove those impediments (work enhancers, WAS-E).

By completing the WAS, people who have MS can describe how the following factors impede their ability to complete work (WAS-I): impairments in mobility, hand functioning, cognitive functioning, and general body state; and the existence of pain, environmental barriers, or jobs that require heavy labor. The seven factors of the work impediment scale have theta reliability coefficients (a measure of consistency among items within a particular factor or scale) ranging from 0.71 to 0.90 and demonstrate expectable concurrent validity relationships with subscales from measures of daily living skills and symptoms of MS (34).

Valuable for suggesting interventions to increase people's capacities to function in career roles, information from the WAS-E scale helps to determine whether changes are needed in areas such as environmental or job modifications, level of social support, beneficial health practices, and personal attributes and strengths. Internal consistency of the WAS-E subscales was acceptable, with theta coefficients ranging from 0.66 (Healthful Practices) to 0.81 (Personal Attributes). Over a 2- to 3-week period, test-retest correlation coefficients ranged from 0.68 to 0.82. Again, evidence of concurrent validity for the WAS-E occurred in certain expectable relationships between WAS-E subscales and subscales of a daily living scale for people with MS (34). Abstracted from the WAS-E, a sampling of conditions or activities that are considered work enhancing is provided in Table 3.1.

TABLE 3.1: WORK ADJUSTMENT SCALE-E

Sample Enhancing Conditions and Activities

Job Adjustment

    Sit-down job

    Plan tasks when energy is highest

Environmental Adjustment/Adaptive Devices

    Adaptive equipment/devices

    Conveniently arranged supplies

Support

    Emotional support

    Assistance with tasks

Personal Attributes

    Positive attitude

    Control of stress

Personal Health Habits

    Good night's sleep

    Peaceful atmosphere

Source: Selected from Work Enhancement Scale-E (34).

As Gulick (34) noted, the WAS has a number of possible applications in the assessment of people with MS. When used in combination by health and rehabilitation professionals, the WAS-I and WAS-E result in identification not only of work impediments but also of strategies to reduce or remove those impediments. The identification of barriers alone (WAS-I) is obviously only a first step toward helping people with MS perform more effectively in areas such as personal care, homemaking, and employment (WAS-E). With information from the WAS-E, it is also possible to recommend a multifaceted approach to barrier removal that may require changes in the (a) person's interpretation of the situation; (b) person's health practices with regard to diet, rest, and surroundings; and/or (c) nature of the situational demands that the person must satisfy.

Gulick reported on two other scales of interest in the assessment of MS and its implications for the individual. The 15-item ADL Self-Care Scale (ADL-MS) includes four areas of daily functioning that affect the person's performance in a variety of career roles (34,36,37). The four ADL areas included in the scale are fine and gross motor (eating, dressing, bathing, transfer, walking, and travel), socializing/recreation (activities inside and outside the home), sensory/communication (reading, writing, telephoning), and intimacy (confiding, expressions of love, sexual activity). Scores on the ADL-MS correlated as expected with scales on the WAS (34).

The MS-Related Symptoms Checklist (MS-RS) is another valuable instrument (34,37). By the term *instrument*, psychologists mean the form or device used to measure a particular construct. If assessors wish to gain more detailed information regarding the symptoms that people with MS are experiencing, they can administer the MS-RS. Covering a variety of symptoms (26 in all), the MS-RS consists of five factors (symptom clusters) that include 22 of the 26 symptoms measured. The five symptom clusters are termed *motor*, *brainstem*, *mental*, *emotions*, and *elimination*, with the number of items in each factor ranging from three to five (Table 3.2). As was the case with the ADL-MS, scores on the MS-RS correlated as expected with the WAS. Additionally, scores on both measures revealed significant negative changes over a 5-year time period for people with MS, particularly for people who had been diagnosed more recently (37).

Similar in focus to the MS-RS (34), the Multiple Sclerosis Impact Scale (MSIS) (29,38) is an instrument for assessing an individual's physical and psychological status with respect to MS. The MSIS-29 consists of 29 items generated from information provided by 1,530 individuals with MS randomly selected from the Multiple Sclerosis Society membership database in England. The instrument assesses the physical (20 items) and psychological (9 items) impact of MS with high levels of internal consistency (0.80 or better in two samples) and test-retest reliability (0.87). Preceded by the phrase "In the past two weeks, how much have you been bothered by...," physical status items include questions related to balance, mobility, tremors, spasms, and stiffness. Prefaced by the previous introductory phrase, psychological items address topics such as feelings of anxiousness, tension, lack of confidence, and depression. Scores on the MSIS-29 correlated as expected with other measures of functioning, health quality of life, and general health.

Devins et al. (12) reported on the development of another reliable and valid illness intrusiveness measure pertinent to MS, the Illness Intrusiveness Ratings Scale (IIRS). The scale measures the extent to which the person appraises MS as a stressful event that interferes with activities in the following important life domains: relationships and personal development, intimacy, and instrumental activities. Total and subscale

TABLE 3.2: MS-RELATED SYMPTOMS SCALE (MS-RS) SYMPTOM CLUSTERS

Motor	*Sensory*
Arm and leg weakness	Pain
Spasms	Burning
Tremors	Numbness
Knee locking	Pins and needles
Balance problems	*Mental-Emotions*
Falling	Loneliness
Brainstem	Depression
Double and blurred vision	Anxiety
Difficulty swallowing	*Elimination*
Forgetfulness	Urine frequency: day and night
	Trouble making toilet: day and night

Source: Ref. 37.

scores provide valuable information regarding the health care needs of women and men with MS and the interventions needed to minimize illness intrusiveness and enhance psychosocial adaptation. High internal consistency coefficients were reported, and data support the use of both total and scale scores in research. Some research (39) suggests that MS is even more intrusive in these life areas than other chronic conditions such as rheumatoid arthritis and end-stage renal disease. Consequently, vocational planning with adults with MS must involve an assessment of self-perceived symptom severity and the intrusiveness of those symptoms in life role functioning.

Work Role Performance

Power and Hershenson (8) described the initial impact of disability as affecting the work competencies of the individual. The negative impact of an adventitious disability such as MS on work competencies radiates to other aspects of the person such as self-image and work goals. Hence, instruments are needed to determine how a disability affects the work-related competencies of the person and other directly relevant variables such as job mastery and job satisfaction, all of which have a bearing on work role performance. Gulick's Work Assessment Scale (WAS) (34) is useful in this regard, as is the Work Experience Survey, another measure that combines the trait/factor and ecological assessment orientations of this chapter.

The Work Experience Survey

The Work Experience Survey (WES) (19) is a structured interview that enables rehabilitation professionals to determine where MS has created work-related barriers. These barriers may limit the person's capacity to gain access to the worksite, perform essential functions, and/or maintain job mastery and satisfaction. Research with the WES clarifies both the types of barriers faced in the workplace and the accommodations used to reduce or remove those barriers (40,41). Evidence also suggests that the number of barriers in the areas of (a) access and performance of essential functions and (b) job mastery have a significant inverse relationship with level of job satisfaction (42).

In completing the WES interview with a rehabilitation professional, the person with MS identifies not only barriers to productivity but also the accommodations needed to reduce or remove those barriers. With information from the WES, individuals are in a position to direct their own accommodation planning consistent with employment provisions and protections in Title I of the Americans with Disabilities Act (ADA; see Chapter 5). Administered in a face-to-face or telephone interview by a rehabilitation professional, the WES consists of six sections: (a) background information on the respondent, (b) an accessibility checklist, (c) an essential job functions checklist, (d) a job mastery survey, (e) a job satisfaction survey, and (f) an accommodation plan.

The accommodation plan describes how techniques such as job restructuring, worksite modification, and/or the addition of new technology would enable the person to maintain productivity on the job. Information from the sections of the WES, described below, is necessary if the rehabilitation professional is to prepare a thorough case study describing the factors that positively and negatively affect job retention for the person with MS (42,43).

ASSESSING ACCESSIBILITY. Adapted from a checklist published by the President's Committee on Employment of People with Disabilities (44), the accessibility section addresses barriers that the worker may experience in entering the worksite, using necessary services and facilities, and exiting the worksite in emergency situations (Table 3.3). If an accessibility issue is not in the checklist, a space is provided for the respondent to list additional accessibility problems. The final question asks the person to describe solutions for his or her two most important accessibility barriers.

TABLE 3.3: ASSESSING ACCESSIBILITY

Section II. Accessibility: Check any problems you have getting to, from, or around on your job. List any other accessibility problems not included in the list. Describe solutions for your two most important accessibility barriers.

___ Parking	___ Bathrooms	___ Temperature
___ Public walks	___ Water Fountains	___ Ventilation
___ Passenger loading zones	___ Public telephone	___ Hazards
___ Entrance	___ Elevators	___ Identification signs/labels
___ Stairs/Steps	___ Lighting	___ Access to personnel offices
___ Floors/Floor covering	___ Warning Devices	___ Access to general use areas
___ Seating/Tables	___ Evacuation routes	

List any other accessibility problems:

#1 _____

_____

#2 _____

_____

Describe solutions for your two most important accessibility barriers.

#1 _____

_____

#2 _____

_____

_____

ASSESSING ESSENTIAL JOB FUNCTIONS. Adapted from the RehabMatch program, Department of Labor research (45), and recommendations from employment specialists familiar with MS and other severe disabilities, the section on essential job functions is divided into six categories: physical abilities, cognitive abilities, task-related abilities, social abilities, working conditions, and company policies (Table 3.4). This section enables the person to check any essential job functions, working conditions, or company policies that constitute problems. The final question in the section asks the individual to describe two potentially helpful accommodations. These accommodations might involve one or more of the strategies suggested in Title I of the ADA, such as restructuring of existing facilities, restructuring of the job, modification of work schedules, reassignment to other positions, modification of existing equipment, installation of new equipment, flexible personal leave policies, provision of qualified readers or interpreters, and modification of application and

51

TABLE 3.4: ASSESSING ESSENTIAL FUNCTIONS

Section III. Essential job functions: Check any essential job functions or conditions* that pose problems for you. Describe the two most important job modifications that you need; e.g., modifying existing equipment, adding new technology, or changing the type of work you do.

Physical Abilities

____ Working 8 hours
____ Standing all day
____ Standing part of the time
____ Walking for 8 hours
____ Some kneeling
____ Some stooping
____ Some climbing
____ Much pulling
____ Much pushing
____ Much talking
____ Seeing well
____ Hearing well
____ Handling
____ Raising arms above shoulders
____ Using both hands
____ Using both legs
____ Using left hand
____ Using right hand
____ Using left leg
____ Using right leg

Cognitive Abilities

____ Immediate memory
____ Short-term memory
____ Judgment: safety
____ Judgment: interpersonal
____ Thought processing
____ Reasoning
____ Problem solving
____ Planning
____ Organizing

Task Related Abilities

____ Repetitive work
____ Work pace/sequencing
____ Variety of duties
____ Perform under stress/deadlines
____ Little feedback on performance
____ Read written instructions
____ Able and licensed to drive
____ Attain precise standards/limits
____ Follow specific instructions
____ Writing

Social Abilities

____ Working alone
____ Working around others
____ Long-term memory
____ Short-term memory
____ Interacting with supervisors
____ Supervision of others
____ Working with hostile others

Working Conditions

____ Too hot
____ Too cold
____ Temperature changes
____ Too wet
____ Too humid
____ Slippery surfaces
____ Obstacles in path
____ Dust
____ Fumes
____ Odors
____ Noise
____ Outdoors

___ Lifting over 100 lb
___ Lifting 51–100 lb
___ Lifting 26–50 lb
___ Lifting 11–25 lb
___ Lifting 0–10 lb
___ Prolonged sitting

___ Remembering
___ Speaking /Communicating
___ Initiating work activities
___ Use sick time

___ Sometimes outdoors
___ Always inside

Company Policies

___ Inflexible work schedules
___ No accrual of sick leave
___ Lack of flextime
___ No "comp" time
___ Inflexible job descriptions
___ Vague job descriptions
___ Infrequent reviews of job descriptions
___ Rigid sick/vacation leave policies

Describe the two job modifications that would be most helpful to you; e.g., restructuring of the job, modification of work schedules, reassignment to another position, modification of equipment, or provision of readers and interpreters.

#1 _____

#2 _____

Source: Adapted from *RehabMatch.* Arkansas Research and Training Center in Vocational Rehabilitation.

examination procedures (17). For example, problems encountered in performing essential functions involving cognitive operations (e.g., memory) could be resolved if individuals dictated notes from meetings using a hand-held recorder, used e-mail messages to themselves for personal reminders, or used an electronic device such as a personal digital assistant to record commitments (46). Mobility limitations become less problematic if the person's desk computer is linked to an electronic mail system. Finally, a flexible work schedule that allows the person to rest during the work day and work later in the evening is an effective response to the fatigue associated with MS.

Assessing Job Mastery

The job mastery scale (coefficient alpha = 0.74) (42) was adapted from *The Career Mastery Inventory* (CMI) developed by John Crites (47). In addition to providing his permission for the use of the items, Crites determined that the content of the items was appropriate for assessing job mastery concerns. The abbreviated measure includes items representing the six domains of *The Career Mastery Inventory:* getting the job done, fitting into the workplace, learning the ropes, getting along with others, getting ahead, and planning the next career step. At the close of the section, the respondent is asked to describe one solution for each of his or her two top priority job mastery concerns (Table 3.5).

Assessing Job Satisfaction

Presented in Table 3.6, the job satisfaction checklist (coefficient alpha = 0.78; [42]) was adapted from the Minnesota Theory of Work Adjustment (26,33). Respondents evaluate their satisfaction with their current jobs in terms of the 20 work reinforcers in the Minnesota theory. An example of the work reinforcer "I do things that make use of my abilities" may be responded to in one of three ways: (a) too little, (b) about right, or (c) too much. Respondents complete the section by listing two ways to make their jobs more personally satisfying. The changes identified may require discussing strategies for either decreasing or increasing the presence of a given reinforcer on the job.

PREPARING AN ACCOMMODATION PLAN. To conclude the WES, respondents select their three highest priority barriers, suggest reasonable accommodations for those barriers, and indicate who could help implement reasonable accommodations and how they could help

(Table 3.7). The information collected in this section of the WES constitutes the essential elements of an accommodation plan that the person can share with his or her employer. In presenting information in the accommodation plan to the employer, the respondent should emphasize the relationship between barrier removal and increased productivity.

ADMINISTERING THE WES. Rehabilitation professionals may administer the WES in a face-to-face (41,43) or telephone interview (40) with individuals with disabilities who are either employed or about to begin employment. Whether conducted by telephone or in person, the WES interview requires 30 to 60 minutes to complete. Face-to-face contact enables the administrator to elicit more information from the respondent because it provides greater opportunity for feelings of trust to develop and for clarification of responses. Prior to administering the WES, rehabilitation professionals may wish to mentally "walk through" the interview using their own jobs as models.

The general procedure for completing the WES Sections II through V is as follows:

1. Engage the person in identifying barriers to accessibility, performance of essential functions, job mastery, and job satisfaction.
2. Ask the person if any problems were overlooked; that is, not included in the checklist. If so, record the additional barriers in the appropriate section.
3. Encourage the person to suggest reasonable accommodations for the barriers; do not hesitate to share knowledge of accommodations that might prove feasible in the person's employment setting.
4. Help the person complete Section VI based on a thorough review of information in the preceding sections of the WES.
5. Remind the person that Section VI constitutes the basis for initiating a review of accommodation needs with the employer. It enables the person to state barriers to productivity in priority order, reasonable accommodation options for each barrier, and potential resources that could assist in barrier removal.

The WES administrator should make every effort to encourage respondents to elaborate on their impressions of their work environments, job duties, and barriers to their productivity. Such information is particularly useful when the rehabilitation professional is not familiar with the job that the person performs. For example, the WES administrator

TABLE 3.5: ASSESSING JOB MASTERY

Section IV. Job Mastery: Check any concerns that affect your success in completing the following tasks. Describe one solution for each of your two most important concerns.

1. Getting the job done
   - ___ Believing that others think I do a good job.
   - ___ Understanding how my job fits into the "big picture"; i.e., the meaning of my job.
   - ___ Knowing what I need to know to do my job.
   - ___ Having what I need to do my job (knowledge, tools, supplies, equipment).

2. Fitting into the workforce
   - ___ Scheduling and planning my work ahead of time.
   - ___ Working mostly because I like the job.
   - ___ Doing a good job.
   - ___ Willing to make changes when necessary.

3. Learning the ropes
   - ___ Knowing who to go to if I need help.
   - ___ Understanding company rules and regulations.
   - ___ Knowing my way around work.
   - ___ Feeling a "part" of what is going on at work.

4. Getting along with others
   - ___ Eating lunch with friends at work.
   - ___ Having many friends at work.
   - ___ Looking forward to seeing my friends at work.
   - ___ Knowing what is expected of me socially on the job.

5. Getting ahead
   - ___ Having a plan for where I want to be in my job in the future.
   - ___ Understanding what I have to do to get promoted.
   - ___ Knowing what training to complete to improve chances for promotion.
   - ___ Talking with supervisor about what I need to do to get promoted.

6. Planning the next career step
   - ___ Considering what I will do in the future.
   - ___ Knowing what the opportunities are in this company.
   - ___ Wanting to become more specialized in my job.
   - ___ Having a good idea of how to advance in this company.

Describe one solution for each of your two most important job mastery concerns.

#1 _____

#2 _____

Source: Selected items from *The Career Mastery Inventory*. Used with permission of the author, John O. Crites, Crites Career Consultants, Boulder, CO.

TABLE 3.6: ASSESSING JOB SATISFACTION

Section V. Satisfaction: Rate your current job on each of the following statements. Describe two ways to make your job more personally satisfying.

In my job . . . (check one)	Too Little	About Right	Too Much
I do things that make use of my abilities.	—	—	—
The job gives me a feeling of accomplishment.	—	—	—
I am busy all the time.	—	—	—
I can work alone on the job.	—	—	—
I do something different everyday.	—	—	—
My pay compares well with that of other workers.	—	—	—
The job provides for steady employment.	—	—	—
The job has good working conditions.	—	—	—
The job provides an opportunity for advancement.	—	—	—
I get recognition for the work I do.	—	—	—
I tell people what to do.	—	—	—
I am "somebody" in the community.	—	—	—
My coworkers are easy to make friends with.	—	—	—
I can do the work without feeling it is morally wrong.	—	—	—
I can do things for other people.	—	—	—
The company administers its policies fairly.	—	—	—
My boss backs up the workers with top management.	—	—	—
My boss trains the workers well.	—	—	—
I try out some of my ideas.	—	—	—
I make my decisions on my own.	—	—	—

Describe two ways to make your job more personally satisfying.

#1 _____

#2 _____

Source: Work reinforcers from Minnesota Theory of Work Adjustment. Dawis, R. & Lofquist, L. (1984). *A psychological theory of work adjustment.* Minneapolis: University of Minnesota.

57

TABLE 3.7: DEVELOPING AN ACCOMMODATION PLAN

Section VI. Review Sections II–V of the WES and list the three most significant barriers to success in your work. Describe their solutions and people/resources who can help. Be specific.

Barrier 1: _____

_____

_____

Solution? _____

_____

_____

Who can help ? How can they help? _____

_____

Barrier 2: _____

_____

_____

Solution? _____

_____

_____

Who can help? How can they help? _____

_____

Barrier 3: _____

_____

_____

Solution? _____

_____

_____

Who can help? How can they help? _____

_____

may not understand the details when a person states that she is an assembler. One respondent who worked on an assembly line used an air gun to place cover-boot wire around control panels on washing machines. Clearly, most WES administrators would need to ask additional information to understand the demands of this task.

Respondents may also have difficulty discriminating between their job *titles* and their job *duties*. For example, a public school teacher needs to consider specific teaching functions and any barriers encountered in performing those functions. Essential functions of the teaching process include tasks such as reading, grading, talking/lecturing, writing, supervising children's activities, and attending faculty meetings. Even functions such as supervision and lecturing can be broken down into more specific tasks.

Throughout the administration of the WES, the interviewer should explain the meaning of any terms that are unfamiliar. For example, cognitive items in the essential functions section may require clarification. Respondents may question what temperature and ventilation have to do with accessibility. The interviewer should explain that excessive heat or cold or poor air circulation could influence one's breathing, which in turn affects mobility.

Some respondents have also requested clarification in responding to items in the job satisfaction section (Section V). The administrator should instruct respondents to consider all items in relationship to the concept of job satisfaction. For example, in presenting the item "I do something different every day," the administrator should ask, "Are you satisfied with this?" If the respondent answers "yes," the correct answer is "about right." If the respondent says "no," the correct response is one that indicates dissatisfaction; that is, "too little" or "too much." The interviewer must probe to determine whether the person does "too little" or "too much" of the same thing every day.

Parts of the WES such as Sections II, III, and VI are helpful for unemployed people with MS who are planning to return to work. Information in the WES can help them identify suitable types of jobs and work environments and the assistive devices/accommodations they might need. They can also consider community agencies, technology resources, and employer-based services that are available to assist them in resuming work. Using the WES for prospective employment is basically a "needs" assessment; for example, how accessible would the worksite have to be, how warm or cool would the work area have to be, could job duties involve walking long distances, what types of accommodations would be needed, and what resources are available.

The WES is also helpful for people with MS who have not disclosed their condition and have some discomfort about the prospect of disclosure. The WES can help them focus on concrete information, involve them in constructive problem-solving activities, and assist them in identifying appropriate people and agencies for resources. This type of focusing, and the resulting knowledge, may lessen their concerns about disclosure (48).

The Goldberg Scale

The Goldberg Scale addresses the theme of psychological uncertainty, which often stands as the greatest barrier to the resumption and retention of work for people with MS. Assessing the construct of vocational development, the Goldberg Scale measures problems encountered by people with disabilities that have a bearing on their motivation to work, vocational realism, and rehabilitation outlook. This information is gathered by asking the respondent to answer a series of "semi-structured questions that elicit a person's vocational plans, interests, work values, motivation to work, and rehabilitation outlook" (9).

Administered in two stages, each interview requires approximately 1 hour to complete. Raters review the person's answers to arrive at an estimate of the individual's rehabilitation outlook, which includes motivation to return to work, a realistic assessment of capacities and physical limitations, and optimism about future recovery and rehabilitation after treatment.

Scores on the Goldberg Scale provide important insights into the probability that a person will successfully complete a rehabilitation program. People with a negative rehabilitation outlook have a low probability of success and experience feelings of hopelessness and devastation. Motivation to return to work, realistic assessment of capacities, and optimism are predictive of successful return to work. Because these factors play at least as important a role in resumption of employment as severity of disability, the rehabilitation professional should consider assessing and intervening in vocational development for individuals with MS who have not succeeded in resuming or retaining employment.

Applications

The assessments presented in this chapter have many applications. First, they are extremely useful in the counseling relationship because they provide valuable information regarding both person and environment factors that affect vocational success. For example, data on work reinforcer preferences, vocational interests, type and seriousness of MS symptoms, and past work history are pertinent to determining whether individuals will be successful in a current or prior line of work or whether they should pursue a related but different type of job. Information on rehabilitation outlook and self-care behaviors provides insights into the extent to which the person is likely to complete a rehabilitation program as well as to maintain a healthy lifestyle. Finally, findings regarding barriers in the work environment that require accommodation or modification are directly relevant to the person's chances to secure and retain desirable employment.

Findings from the assessments described in this chapter are useful to disability management professionals who seek to improve the employment-related services of employers. The purposes of disability management interventions are both to ensure the rapid return of well-trained, loyal workers to the workplace following injury and to help employers contain the rising costs of disability and health care (18). Information from assessments such as the WAS-I, WAS-E, and WES help employer and employee to collaborate in identifying barriers to productivity and cost-effective accommodations. Cost-effective (reasonable) accommodations can control rising workers' compensation and health care costs, which are consuming an increasing share of employer resources (49). One should also note that the assessments described in this chapter are not only for employees with MS or even other types of disabilities, but also for other major segments of today's work force such as older workers. By gathering information pertinent to helping people care for themselves and remain productive at work, employers can retain trained workers during a time when decreasing numbers of workers with adequate skills are available in the labor market (50).

The Relevance of Assessments in the Americans with Disabilities Act

Information from assessments that identify factors affecting a person's capacity to do work is extremely relevant in the ADA era. Title I of the ADA describes employment protections that require accommodations of employees with disabilities so that they can perform essential job functions, provided that the accommodations do not constitute an undue hardship for the employer (51,52). Data from the WAS-I, WAS-E, and WES are useful throughout the accommodation process prescribed by the ADA to resolve problems that people with MS face in performing their jobs. Feldblum (53) described the steps of the accommodation process as follows:

1. The employee or applicant may initiate the request for an accommodation, to which the employer is required to respond.
2. The individual and the employer collaborate in a process of identifying the barriers that limit the worker's abilities to perform essential functions of the job.
3. Using the person with a disability as a source of information, the employer identifies a variety of accommodations.
4. The employer assesses the cost effectiveness of each of the accommodations to determine which ones can be made with the least economic hardship to the business.
5. The employer implements the most appropriate accommodation with due consideration of the person's preferences in the case of two or more accommodations deemed equal in cost effectiveness.

Information from the WES can help employees understand specifically what their work limitations are, the priority to place on those limitations, and examples of reasonable accommodations (46). This information is useful throughout the five steps of the accommodation process. Moreover, the WES enables the employer to involve the person with a disability in the accommodation process, as Feldblum (53) suggested in step 3.

Assessment Data and Limiting the Intrusiveness of Disability

Ranging from measures of concrete constructs such as symptoms and daily living skills to more abstract concepts such as rehabilitation outlook, the assessments described in this chapter provide information regarding potentially helpful strategies to reduce the intrusiveness of MS and other severe disabilities. In addition to their physical effects, chronic illnesses and severe disabilities such as MS are intrusive psychological stressors that increase role strain, disrupt economic and vocational stability, and create a sense of helplessness and external control (6,54,55).

Understanding how MS has affected them can help people assume a more empowered role in the rehabilitation process. As a result, they gain a greater sense of self-efficacy, the belief that they have the power to achieve desirable outcomes and avoid negative ones (56). Experiences that enhance self-efficacy are desirable antidotes to the negative impact of disability and chronic illness on personal control.

Summary

Several basic premises underlie this chapter on assessment of the employment needs of people with MS. For example, the strategy of least intervention may be the most sensible: that is, assist the person in retaining employment in the same job with the same employer. If this is not possible, the person may initiate and direct his or her own vocational analysis with some assistance and identify related vocational roles that are available in the local job market. Occupational information resources such as the O*NET, *Guide for Occupational Exploration,* and the *Occupational Outlook Handbook* are useful in this effort, as are specific assessments such as the Minnesota Importance Questionnaire (MIQ) and the Minnesota Satisfactoriness Scales (MSS).

Two other premises in the chapter work hand in hand; that is, the concept of career development is more encompassing than simply functioning in vocational roles, and both person and environment must be assessed to identify appropriate vocational placements. Measures of symptoms associated with MS (MS-RS, MSIS-29) and factors impeding or enhancing the capacity to work at home, in the community, and in one's job (ADL-MS, WAS-I, and WAS-E) operationalize a broader and more useful career construct. With information from these measures and other types of assessments such as job analyses, the rehabilitation professional can determine which person and environment interventions have the potential of maximizing the person's capacity to do work: that is, to expend energy to achieve personal goals in a wide range of settings.

By concentrating specifically on workplace barriers, the Work Experience Survey (WES) addresses the problem of excessively high unemployment rates among people with MS. The WES is based on the assumption that barriers may occur in four areas: access to the workplace, performance of essential functions, job mastery, and job satisfaction. Problems identified in any of the four areas are responsive to on-the-job adjustments ranging from the use of technology and other accommodative strategies to the changing of certain company policies or supervisory techniques. Suggested job accommodations and information as to who can assist the individual and how they can assist are organized in an accommodation plan for the final section of the WES.

Goldberg's measure of vocational development is useful for those individuals with MS who are having difficulty coping with the psychological uncertainty of the illness and its debilitating effects on the resumption and/or retention of employment. With its emphasis on motivation, realism, and optimism, the Goldberg Scale provides valuable insights into the person's rehabilitation outlook, a variable that research has shown to be related to work resumption. Scores on this scale may help the rehabilitation professional determine the types of psychological problems that the person is experiencing and the interventions that have the greatest potential to restore the person's motivation to continue employment.

Throughout all of the discussion of the various measurement strategies, the reader should keep in mind the broad applications related to the assessment of people with MS. Accurate assessment information on factors impeding and enhancing the production of work (defined broadly) can help (a) employers improve their disability management services, (b) people with MS participate in and benefit from the accommodation protections in the ADA, and (c) people with MS and their families take control of the rehabilitation and accommodation process in order to counter the helplessness and depression that are frequently experienced in coping with the impact of chronic illness and disability.

References

1. LaRocca, N. (1995). *Employment and multiple sclerosis.* New York: National Multiple Sclerosis Society.
2. Rao, S., Leo, G., Ellington, L., et al. (1991). Cognitive dysfunction in multiple sclerosis: Impact on employment and social functioning. *Neurology, 41*(5), 692–696.
3. Roessler, R., Fitzgerald, S., Rumrill, P., & Koch, L. (2001). Determinant of employment status among people with multiple sclerosis. *Rehabilitation Counseling Bulletin, 45,* 31–39.
4. Roessler, R., Rumrill, P., & Fitzgerald, S. (2004). Predictors of employment status for people with multiple sclerosis. *Rehabilitation Counseling Bulletin, 47,* 96–103.
5. Falvo, D. (2005). *Medical and psychological aspects of chronic illness and disability.* 3rd Edition. Sudberry, MA: Jones and Bartlett.
6. Roessler, R. (2004). The illness intrusiveness model: Rehabilitation implications. *Journal of Applied Rehabilitation Counseling, 35*(3), 22–27.
7. LaRocca, N., Kalb, R., Scheinberg, L., & Kendall, P. (1985). Factors associated with unemployment of patients with multiple sclerosis. *Journal of Chronic Diseases, 38,* 203–210.

8. Power, P., & Hershenson, D. (2001). Assessment of career development and maturity. In B. Bolton (Ed.), *Handbook of measurement and evaluation in rehabilitation*. 3rd Edition. Gaithersburg, MD: Aspen, pp. 339–364.

9. Goldberg, R. (1992). Toward a model of vocational development of people with disabilities. *Rehabilitation Counseling Bulletin, 35*, 161–173.

10. Rounds, J., & Armstrong, P. (2005). Assessment of needs and values. In S. Brown & R. Lent (Eds.), *Career development andcCounseling*. New York: John Wiley, pp. 305–329.

11. Stanford Patient Education Research Center. (2007). Adapted Illness Intrusiveness Ratings. Retrieved 4/9/07, www. patienteducation.stanford.edu/research/illnessintrusiveness.html.

12. Devins, G., Dion, R., Pelletier, L., et al. (2001). Structure and lifestyle disruptions in chronic disease: a confirmatory factor analysis of the illness Intrusiveness Ratings Scale. *Medical Care, 39*(10), 1097–1104.

13. Dawis, R. (2002). Person-environment-correspondence theory. In D. Brown and Associates (Eds.), *Career choice and development*. 4th Edition. San Francisco, CA: Jossey-Bass, pp. 427–464.

14. Hershenson, D. (1992). A theoretical model for rehabilitation counseling. *Rehabilitation Counseling Bulletin, 33*, 268–278.

15. Kosciulek, J. (1993). Advances in trait-and-factor theory: A person-environment approach to rehabilitation counseling. *Journal of Applied Rehabilitation Counseling, 24*(2), 11–14.

16. Dobren, A. (1994). An ecologically oriented conceptual model of vocational rehabilitation of people with acquired mid-career disabilities. *Rehabilitation Counseling Bulletin, 37*, 215–228.

17. Roessler, R., & Rubin, S. (2006). Rehabilitation counseling and case management. Austin: PRO-ED.

18. Brodwin, M. (2001). Rehabilitation in the private-for-profit sector: Opportunities and challenges. In S. Rubin & R. Roessler (Eds.), *Foundations of the vocational rehabilitation process*. 5th Edition. Austin, TX: PRO-ED, pp. 475–496.

19. Roessler, R. (1995). *The work experience survey*. Fayetteville: Arkansas Research and Training Center in Vocational Rehabilitation.

20. Power, P. (2006). Operationalizing the concept of empowerment during the vocational assessment process. *Journal of Applied Rehabilitation Counseling, 37*, 21–25.

21. O*NET (2007). Retrieved 4/30/07 from www. online.onetcenter.org.

22. Farr, J., Ludden, L., and Shatkin, L. (2001). *The guide for occupational exploration*. Indianapolis: JIST.

23. *Occupational outlook handbook* (2007). Retrieved 4/21/07 from www.bls.gov/OCO.

24. Farr, J., & Ludden, L. (2003). *Enhanced occupational outlook*. Indianapolis: JIST.

25. U.S. Department of Labor (2007). Retrieved 4/13/07 from www.dol.gov.

26. Dawis, R. (2005). The Minnesota theory of work adjustment. In S. Brown & R. Lent (Eds.), *Career development and counseling*. New York: John Wiley, pp. 3–23.

27. Parker, R., Szymanski, E., & Hanley-Maxwell, C. (1989). Ecological assessment in supported employment. *Journal of Applied Rehabilitation Counseling, 20*(3), 26–33.

28. Kornblith, A., LaRocca, N., & Baum, H. (1986). Employment in individuals with multiple sclerosis. *International Journal of Rehabilitation Research, 9*, 155–165.

29. Larsen, P. (1990). Psychosocial adjustment in multiple sclerosis. *Rehabilitation Nursing, 15*(5), 242–247.

30. Patterson, J. (2003). Occupational and labor market information: Resources and application. In E. Szymanski & R. Parker (Eds.), *Work and disability*. 2nd Edition. Austin: PRO-ED, pp. 247–280.

31. LaRocca, N., & Hall, H. (1990). Multiple sclerosis program: A model for neuropsychiatric disorders. *New Directions for Mental Health Services, 45,* 49–64.
32. Minnesota Importance Questionnaire (2007). Retrieved 4/10/07 from www.psych. umn.edu/psylabs/vpr/miqinf.htm.
33. Dawis, R. & Lofquist, L. (1984). *A psychological theory of work adjustment.* Minneapolis: University of Minnesota Press.
34. Gulick, E. (1991). Reliability and validity of the Work Assessment Scale for persons with multiple sclerosis. *Nursing Research, 40,* 107–112.
35. Gulick, E. (1992). Model for predicting work performance among persons with multiple sclerosis. *Nursing Research, 41*(5), 266–272.
36. Gulick, E. (1987). Parsimony and model confirmation of the ADL Self-Care Scale for people with multiple sclerosis. *Nursing Research, 36,* 278–283.
37. Gulick, E., & Bugg, A. (1992). Holistic health patterning in multiple sclerosis. *Research in Nursing & Health, 15,* 175–185.
38. Hobart, J., Lamping, D., Fitzpatrick, et al. (2001). The Multiple Sclerosis Impact Scale (MSIS-29). *Brain, 124,* 962–973.
39. Devins, G., Edworthy, S., Seland, T., et al. (1993). Differences in illness intrusiveness across rheumatoid arthritis, end-stage renal disease, and multiple sclerosis. *Journal of Nervous and Mental Disease, 181*(6), 377–381.
40. Allaire, S., Wei, L., & LaValley, M. (2003). Work barriers experienced and job accommodations used by persons with arthritis and other rheumatic diseases. *Rehabilitation Counseling Bulletin, 46*(3), 147–156.
41. Allaire, S., Niu, J., & LaValley, M. (2005). Employment and satisfaction outcomes from a job retention intervention. *Rehabilitation Counseling Bulletin, 48*(2), 100–109.
42. Roessler, R., & Rumrill, P. (1995). The relationship of perceived worksite barriers to job mastery and job satisfaction for employed people with multiple sclerosis. *Rehabilitation Counseling Bulletin, 39*(1), 2–14.
43. Roessler, R., & Gottcent, J. (1994). The Work Experience Survey: A reasonable accommodation/career development strategy. *Journal of Applied Rehabilitation Counseling, 25*(3), 16–21.
44. President's Committee on Employment of People with Disabilities (1985). *Employers are asking ... about the safety of handicapped workers when emergencies occur.* Washington, DC: U.S. Government Printing Office.
45. Greenwood, R., Johnson, V., Wilson, J., & Schriner, K. (1988). *RehabMatch.* Fayetteville: Arkansas Research and Training Center in Vocational Rehabilitation.
46. Johnson, K. (2006). Disclosure to employer and using job accommodations. In R. Fraser, G. Kraft, D. Ehde, & K. Johnson (Eds.), *The MS workbook.* Oakland, CA: New Harbinger, pp. 105–116.
47. Crites, J. (1990). *The career mastery inventory.* Boulder: Crites Career Consultants.
48. Fraser, R. (2006). Employment strategies and community resources. In R. Fraser, G. Kraft, D. Ehde, & K. Johnson (Eds.), *The MS workbook.* Oakland, CA: New Harbinger, pp. 105–116.
49. Creen, M. (2002). Best practices for disability management. *Journal of the Ontario Occupational Health Nurses Association,* Winter, 5–8.
50. Schramm, J. (2006). SHRM workforce forecast. Alexandria, VA: Society for Human Resource Management.
51. Colker, R. (2005). *The disability pendulum.* New York: New York University Press.
52. Roessler, R., & Rumrill, P. (1995). The Work Experience Survey: A structured interview approach to worksite accommodation planning. *Journal of Job Placement, 11*(1):15–19.

53. Feldblum, C. (1991). Employment protections. In J. West (Ed.), *The Americans with Disabilities Act: From policy to practice*. New York: Milbank Memorial Fund, pp. 81–110.

54. Devins, G., & Seland, T. (1987). Emotional impact of multiple sclerosis: Recent findings and suggestions for future research. *Psychological Bulletin, 101*, 363–375.

55. Devins, G., & Shnek, Z. (2000). Multiple sclerosis. In R. Frank & T. Elliot (Eds.), *Handbook of rehabilitation psychology*. Washington, DC: American Psychological Association, pp.163–184.

56. Bandura, A. (1986). Social foundations of thought and action: *A social cognitive theory*. Englewood Cliffs, NJ: Prentice-Hall.

57. Rumrill, P. (1996). Employment issues and multiple sclerosis. New York: Demos Vermande.

58. Schwartz, G., Watson, S., Galvin, D., & Lipoff, E. (1989). *The disability management sourcebook*. Washington, DC: Washington Business Group on Health and Institute for Rehabilitation and Disability Management.

Employment and Career Development Interventions

Steven W. Nissen

Phillip D. Rumrill, Jr.

Mary L. Hennessey

O NCE THE INTERESTS, APTITUDES, functional abilities, health status, and work experience of a person with multiple sclerosis (MS) have been assessed using instruments and procedures such as those described in Chapter 3, attention turns to the services, supports, and assistance that he or she may need to resume or continue his or her career while coping with MS. Help is available! Over the past 30 years, there has emerged a wealth of resources, demonstration projects, research, direct services, and advocacy efforts to promote the employment and career advancement of people with MS and other disabling conditions. Some of these interventions are designed specifically for people with MS, and others target people with all types of disabilities. Some of these interventions are delivered by rehabilitation professionals, and others are of the "self-help" variety. Some of these interventions are delivered in person, and others can be accessed via telephone or the Internet. Some of these interventions focus on job acquisition (i.e., getting a job), and others focus on job retention (i.e., keeping and advancing in the job one has).

As different as these programs and projects are in design and implementation, together they form a powerful set of tools and strategies for combating the deleterious impact that MS too often exacts on a person's employment status. In this chapter, we describe the essential elements and outcomes of employment interventions that have proven efficacious or could be helpful to people with MS in their career-related pursuits. We begin by highlighting MS-specific interventions, then we follow with descriptions of several national-scale programs that address the employment needs and concerns of Americans with various disabilities.

MS-Specific Interventions

A number of research, demonstration, and direct service initiatives have been developed in recent years to address the specific employment concerns of people with MS. In no order of priority, scope, or impact, we discuss several of these initiatives in the following pages.

MS Employment Assistance Service: Kent State University

Since 1999, the Center for Disability Studies at Kent State University in Ohio has offered employment assistance and career counseling services to adults with MS [1]. The MS Employment Assistance Service is staffed by nationally Certified Rehabilitation Counselors who provide a wide range of vocational services, including the following:

- Career Counseling
- Assessments of Vocational Interests and Aptitudes
- Transferable Skills Analysis
- Resume Preparation
- Interview Skills Training
- Targeted Job Placement Assistance
- Social Security Advocacy
- Self-Advocacy Training
- Benefits Planning
- Referrals to Legal Resources
- On-the-Job Accommodation Planning
- Consultation in Employment Litigation

All services are provided via telephone or e-mail, and each participant develops a customized plan of services and assistance from the "menu" described above. Some participants use the MS Employment Assistance Service over an extended time period, whereas others call or e-mail for specific, point-in-time answers to employment-related questions and concerns. The service is supported by subscriptions from individual chapters of the National Multiple Sclerosis Society, and 2,411 people with MS representing 16 chapters of the Society have taken part in the project as of this writing (1). The most common employment-related issues raised by people with MS inquiring to the service include job search (46 percent of participants), workplace discrimination and employer relations (42 percent), short- and long-term disability (40 percent), Social Security (38 percent), on-the-job accommodations (37 percent), disclosure of disability (34 percent), the Family and Medical Leave Act (27 percent), and home-based employment (19 percent). The percentages in the preceding list total more than 100 percent because most participants inquire to the MS Employment Assistance Service with more than one issue or concern.

Operation Job Match

Founded in 1980 as a job readiness training program, Operation Job Match (OJM) is the employment assistance and support program of the National Capital Chapter of the National Multiple Sclerosis Society in Washington, DC. As a multiweek employment group, the program addressed a variety of employment- and disability-related issues including job-seeking skills components and a selective placement component. Topics included disability management, stress management, assertiveness training, disclosure issues, accommodation strategies, interview skills, resume and cover letters, and networking. OJM maintained a job bank of positions available in the metropolitan Washington, DC, area and staff then matched program participants to available positions. Job bank participants were private sector employers, federal government agencies, colleges and universities, and nonprofit organizations. Although originally designed for individuals with MS, the program was expanded to include participants with other adult-onset physical disabilities such as lupus, arthritis, diabetes, and spinal cord injury.

Operation Job Match increases the job-seeking proficiency of participants by enlisting assistance from the employer community to generate a wide range of career options. The initial program proved to be so successful that it has been replicated at National Multiple Sclerosis Society chapters throughout the United States. It has also been adopted as a part of the more comprehensive Job Raising Program (2), which is discussed later in this chapter.

Since its creation in 1980, OJM has been the recipient of numerous federal and private grants that have provided the resources to permit the program to change over time. Some federal grants allowed the programs to be replicated across the country. A recent Projects with Industry (PWI) grant from 1997 until 2002 from the United States Department of Education, Rehabilitation Services Administration allowed OJM to focus on telework and alternative work arrangements for people with MS and other significant adult-onset physical disabilities. The project focused on telecommuting, work-at-home, and flexible schedules as an effective means of accommodating the unpredictability and variability of MS and other adult-onset physical conditions. Program funds were available to purchase home office equipment, computer equipment, assistive technology, and assessment and training services. This program had a 53 percent placement rate over the course of the grant, with 72 percent of those placements allowing for some flexibility in the workplace (3). A considerable amount of job development and employer outreach was necessary during this grant-funded program. Finding employers who were receptive to hiring individuals with adult-onset physical disabilities such as MS was critical. Finding employers who were receptive to allowing their employees to work from home or on alternative schedules posed some challenges. Especially with a new employee, the employer was often hesitant to allow that employee to work from home. Therefore, a considerable amount of employer education and support was necessary. In some situations, the employees with MS or other adult-onset physical disability were able to negotiate new positions with their current employers that would allow for more flexibility in the workplace. This worked best when the employees were familiar to the employers, when they were valued and trusted, and when they had the skills to transition smoothly into new positions. This change in work arrangement was also helpful in assisting individuals with job retention and maintaining their employment.

Since the conclusion of the PWI telework program, OJM has continued to provide employment assistance and support under the auspices of the National Capital Chapter of the National Multiple Sclerosis Society. Individual participants work primarily one-on-one with OJM staff to assess their employment needs, assist with managing their disability in the workplace, and determine plans of action to achieve their employment goals. Services can include explanation of legal rights and responsibilities under the Americans with Disabilities Act (ADA), the Family and Medical Leave Act (FMLA), the Health Insurance Portability and Accountability Act (HIPAA), and the Consolidated Omnibus Budget Reconciliation Act

(COBRA); discussing the advantages and disadvantages of disclosing disability status in the workplace; disclosure training; brainstorming practical accommodation strategies; job-seeking skills training including assistance with resumes, cover letters, and interview skills; completion of vocational interest inventories; referral to positions posted through a job bank; referral to and collaboration with other vocational rehabilitation and employment agencies; and follow-along services. In addition to the one-on-one services provided through OJM, periodic training programs are offered in large and small-group settings.

OJM continues to work with the employer community as well. A job bank is available that comprises job vacancy announcements from employers in the metropolitan Washington, DC, area who are turning to OJM in an effort to increase their company's diversity or disability outreach. Announcements come from private industry employers, federal government agencies, colleges and universities, and nonprofit agencies. Job leads are also received by way of other vocational rehabilitation agencies that have distribution lists. For example, a state vocational rehabilitation business development manager may have contact with an employer and receive a lead that is then distributed to service provider agencies that have access to qualified individuals with disabilities. OJM receives such leads as well. OJM staff members review leads as they are received and refer appropriate candidates to apply for the positions.

OJM also conducts in-service trainings to employers. Topics covered include employment issues and MS, employment characteristics of individuals with adult-onset physical conditions, suggestions for working with individuals with invisible disabilities, and how best to supervise someone with MS. Periodic employer programs (e.g., employer breakfasts or lunches) are offered as well to do outreach to a larger employer audience. OJM's employer outreach and input occur through its Business Advisory Committee (BAC). The BAC is primarily comprised of human resource professionals, recruiters, diversity and outreach professionals, and vocational rehabilitation staff. BAC members provide assistance and guidance to OJM related to labor market information, the hiring process, resumes and cover letters, job development, and strategies for hiring OJM clients. They are often recruited as presenters at programs. This is another innovative feature of the Operation Job Match program—incorporating the employer's perspective throughout the employment rehabilitation process.

The Job Raising Program

In 1983, the National Multiple Sclerosis Society, in conjunction with the Arthritis Foundation and a consortium of traumatic brain injury advocacy groups, developed the Job Raising Program. The Job Raising Program represents an employment placement and retention model for people with adult-onset, chronic disabilities. Over an 8-year period, the Job Raising Program assisted a total of 2,338 participants in obtaining and/or maintaining employment. A wide variety of services was provided in a 10-week, small-group (10 to 12 participants) format. Participants received training from community experts on assertiveness, interviewing, resume writing, and labor market trends. Upon completion of the training component, Job Raising participants formed a job search club to provide ongoing support for one another. Job seekers were also introduced to mentors who worked in their chosen fields.

Job Raising proved to be a highly successful program, with 60 percent of all participants (i.e., people with MS, arthritis, and traumatic brain injury) successfully employed at the 8-year follow-up (4). Job Raising participants with MS fared even better than their counterparts with arthritis or brain injuries; 71 percent of these individuals reported being employed at follow-up.

The Career Possibilities Project

The Career Possibilities Project (5) addressed LaRocca's (6) call for empowerment, rights awareness, resource utilization, and community-based services as research priorities concerning the employment of people with MS. Targeting unemployed people with MS in four midwestern cities, the project was designed to increase participants' employment rate, job-seeking activity, employability maturity, optimism about reentering the work force, and career self-efficacy.

Utilizing a two-group, pretest/posttest quasi-experimental design, Rumrill et al. (5) recruited 37 participants from National Multiple Sclerosis Society chapters and MS clinics in the target cities (i.e., Cleveland, OH; Evansville, IN; Louisville, KY; and Milwaukee, WI). Time sampling methods were used to assign the first 23 participants to the Career Possibilities condition and the second 14 participants to the comparison group.

Participants in the comparison group completed a telephone interview with a trained rehabilitation professional about their job-seeking plans.

74

They also received a job-seeking information packet that contained tips and strategies for securing job leads, developing resumes, interviewing, following up after interviews, and networking. The more elaborate Career Possibilities condition included the telephone interview and the Accommodations Planning Team (APT) seminar, which introduced participants to employers in their chosen fields and rehabilitation professionals who could help facilitate the career reentry process. The APT is a half-day program that teaches skills related to (a) identifying prospective accommodation needs; (b) understanding one's legal rights to reasonable accommodations; (c) discussing accommodation needs with employers; and (d) developing resource-directed plans for obtaining career-entry or reentry positions (7).

In the APT seminar, each participant is teamed with an employer and a rehabilitation professional who provide feedback and direction as the person with MS proceeds through the accommodation planning process. The seminar concludes with one member of each team volunteering to contact the participant as a follow-up measure in 2 to 4 weeks.

Results of the Career Possibilities Project revealed that the APT seminar and the less elaborate placement counseling condition (administered to the comparison group) were similarly effective in helping people with MS return to work. From a baseline employment rate of zero, 30 percent (n = 7) of participants in the APT seminar reported being employed at a 16-week follow-up. Twenty-nine percent (n = 4) of the comparison group were also employed at the 4-month checkpoint—thereby supporting Roessler's (8) "least intervention" assertion that unemployed people with MS may need only limited, but focused, assistance to reenter the work force. Overall, the Career Possibilities Project successfully reemployed 11 people with MS who had disengaged from the workforce. With a total budget of $20,000, this project achieved those career reentry outcomes at a very cost-effective rate of $1,818 per placement.

The Progressive Request Model

Rumrill et al. (9) investigated the effects of the Progressive Request Model (PRM) on career maintenance self-efficacy (i.e., confidence in requesting reasonable accommodations), acceptance of disability, and behavioral activity in the ADA's reasonable accommodation process. Participants in the study included 45 employed people with MS who received varying levels of information and training regarding the ADA's accommodation process. Participants were randomly assigned to one of three treatment conditions (i.e., control, prompt, or PRM).

Participants in the control condition received no intervention. Those in the prompt condition completed the Work Experience Survey (WES), a structured needs assessment tool designed to help people with disabilities identify on-the-job accommodations, in a face-to-face interview conducted in their homes. They also received a verbal prompt from the interviewer to approach their employers about their accommodation needs. In the more elaborate PRM condition, participants completed the WES and were provided an ADA self-help guide (10). They were asked to read carefully the guide and be prepared to discuss its contents when the interviewer returned to their homes 1 week later. The second home visit consisted of a review of the guide's contents and a 45-minute social competence training session on how to effectively to request reasonable accommodations from employers.

At an 8-week follow-up, participants in the PRM condition were found to be significantly more confident (i.e., had higher levels of self-efficacy) in their ability to request accommodations than were participants in the control and prompt groups. However, increased self-efficacy was not found to be an antecedent of self-advocacy behaviors such as requests for accommodations made with employers, meetings with employers to discuss accommodations, and accommodations implemented at the worksite; there were no differences among the three groups on those dimensions of accommodation activity (9). Neither were there any differences among the three groups in scores on a short form of the Acceptance of Disability Scale. In speculating as to why this occurred, Rumrill et al. (9) suggested that their micro-skills approach could have limited the overall effectiveness of the intervention. They emphasized the need for employer involvement in all phases of the accommodation planning process—from participation in the WES interview to receiving ADA information and social competence training in making accommodation requests. A brief intervention such as the PRM prompted increased confidence in the accommodation request process, but articulating that confidence into behavioral action probably requires more intensive and longer term training programs. Also important is the involvement of other health professionals (e.g., physical and occupational therapists, nurses, psychologists, physicians, social workers) in helping workers evaluate their functional capacities and then address them through the ADA's accommodation process.

Project Alliance

In 1992, the National Multiple Sclerosis Society introduced Project Alliance, a comprehensive job retention program that combined needs assessment principles (8) and self-advocacy training (9) with employer consultation and community resources. The Project Alliance intervention was made available to employed persons with MS and other adult-onset chronic illnesses at 14 sites nationwide. The 3-year initiative served more than 300 employees and their employers. The primary objectives of this innovative program were:

1. To engage both the employee (with a chronic illness) and the employer in the process of examining the current issues related to job performance.
2. To gather information related to the person's actual position, including the physical and cognitive requirements, the essential and marginal functions, and support systems.
3. To identify barriers to successful job performance.
4. To provide assistance to the employee and the employer in improving communication and in moving toward satisfactory resolution of the (work-related) issues.
5. To assist all parties in understanding the provisions of the ADA and how voluntary compliance can benefit all concerned.
6. To help identify needs of the employee and employer in terms of job modifications, adjustments, or accommodations that could assist the employee in achieving and maintaining satisfactory work performance (11, p. 1).

Project Alliance objectives were achieved by conducting an on-site job analysis that utilized input from the rehabilitation professional, the employee, the employer, and coworkers. The job analyst recorded and interpreted information pertaining to the essential and marginal functions of the position, the employee's general and illness-related health status, the impact of the illness on the employee's job performance, the quality and quantity of the employee's work in comparison to coworkers, on-the-job and community resources that could be consulted, and employee and employer appraisals of the presenting problem(s) (7). The job analyst then synthesized the information into a written report that was presented to both the employee and employer. Finally, follow-along contacts were made to assist in the implementation and monitoring of reasonable accommodations and other job retention strategies.

Because Project Alliance required employees with MS (or other chronic illness) and their employers to work together in the process of identifying, prioritizing, and implementing reasonable accommodations, it exemplifies the ADA's spirit of collaborative decision making and non-adversarial problem solving (see Chapter 5). The project also overcame one of the limitations of the Progressive Request Model intervention by educating employers about the value of retaining experienced and productive employees who may be coping with disabilities but who can still "get the job done."

In general, job retention interventions for people with disabilities are most effective when priority is placed on helping them continue in their present positions (12). The same appears to be true for those with MS, and reasonable accommodations at the worksite constitute a central theme of contemporary MS research and service delivery in the area of career maintenance (9,11,13).

For example, within a sub-sample of successfully employed workers with MS, Kraft et al. (14) noted that the vast majority were employed in the same jobs they had held at the time of diagnosis, and that very few had changed jobs since the onset of their illness. Rumrill (1) asserted that the onset of MS has no effect on a person's vocational interests; it can and does, however, affect a person's ability to continue in his or her chosen field. These findings indicate that rehabilitation services, such as those described in the Progressive Request Model and Project Alliance, should be introduced immediately after diagnosis to assist individuals in keeping their jobs. To be optimally effective, accommodation planning must be tailored to the person's present work environment and job demands. Although a rehabilitation counselor can play a valuable role in identifying accommodation strategies and resources, functional capacities information from medical and allied health professionals is also crucial in the determination of the person's work potential. Moreover, health care professionals are usually people's first point of contact regarding MS, so early referrals to rehabilitation counselors must be made as soon as vocational issues become evident. The "an ounce of prevention is worth a pound of cure" maxim is highly compatible with the mission of job retention services for people with MS, so readers are encouraged to engage career planning interventions as soon after diagnosis as possible.

Career Crossroads: Employment and MS

In 2004, the National Multiple Sclerosis Society produced a comprehensive employment program, *Career Crossroads: Employment and MS*, geared primarily toward individuals who are currently working and hoping to retain employment. This program consists of a video/DVD and accompanying participant manual and leader manual. The program is designed to be implemented in a small-group setting over several weeks. In the video, a fictional character, Claire, is struggling with challenging symptoms that are beginning to affect her job performance as a graphic designer. She has been recently diagnosed but has not disclosed her MS or requested any accommodations. Her friend, fictional character Vanessa, who is a librarian, assists Claire with researching the appropriate steps to request accommodations and tap into available resources in order to maintain her employment. In doing so, actual clients, rehabilitation professionals, attorneys, employers, and medical professionals are interviewed. Topics covered in *Career Crossroads* include:

● The importance of work
● The impact work has on MS and the impact MS has on work
● Legal protections—Americans with Disabilities Act (ADA), Family and Medical Leave Act (FMLA), Health Insurance Portability and Accountability Act (HIPAA), and Consolidated Omnibus Budget Reconciliation Act (COBRA)
● Disclosure—including a disclosure script "formula" and a description of the advantages and disadvantages of disclosing
● Accommodations—practical strategies for managing symptoms in the workplace and the relationship to disclosure
● Resources—including the National Multiple Sclerosis Society, Job Accommodation Network (JAN), United States Equal Employment Opportunity Commission (EEOC), Disability and Business Technical Assistance Centers (DBTAC)
● Information on tax incentives for hiring people with disabilities
● Work-life balance and planning ahead

Each of the six 15-minute segments of the DVD addresses a different topic and the accompanying manual provides factual information on the topic being discussed, exercises to complete and review with the group, and homework assignments. The program is designed to take place over a 7-week period. The intention is that National Multiple Sclerosis Society chapters across the country implement this program. *Career Crossroads* was designed to be a 7-week small group program, but chapters are given the flexibility to offer the program over as many weeks as they choose.

Career Crossroads provides a "program in a box" that can be implemented in a variety of ways. Suggestions are provided in the leader's manual for guest speakers, specific publications and handouts to distribute in each session, and open-ended questions to ask participants.

A self-study, coached version of *Career Crossroads* is available as well. Through this format, participants are provided their own copies of the DVD and an expanded version of the participant manual, which has more exercises to be completed. The program participant schedules regular telephone calls or sessions with a chapter staff member or volunteer familiar with employment issues, who serves as an employment coach. This coach will take the participant through all the segments of *Career Crossroads* at the individual's own pace.

Career Crossroads provides information on a variety of common employment issues for individuals with MS. The intention is for people with MS to become familiar with these issues, know how to handle them if and when they arise in the workplace, and know more about their employment options. This is a way to help individuals with MS to be more confident and knowledgeable in determining ways to retain employment. *Career Crossroads* may also be effective with individuals planning an imminent return to the workplace or considering changing jobs.

Career Crossroads, although originally created for individuals with MS, may be appropriate for people working with other chronic illnesses or disabilities. The program is available from the National Multiple Sclerosis Society for individuals, other nonprofit agencies, and disability agencies that are interested in adapting the program for their own purposes. Contact the National MS Society at www.nationalMSsociety.org or by calling 1-800-344-4867.

MS in the Workplace: A Guide for Employers

In 2007, the National Multiple Sclerosis Society released a DVD entitled *MS in the Workplace: A Guide for Employers*. This video is geared toward employer representatives—human resource professionals, recruiters, diversity outreach professionals, and supervisors and coworkers of people with MS. The underlying message is that hiring and retaining people with MS makes good business sense. It would be a disservice to ignore the talents and contributions that people with MS, and disabilities in general, can bring to the workplace. The video features employees with MS as well as employers discussing the importance of having a diverse work force.

MS in the Workplace: A Guide for Employers contains information regarding some of the key components of the employment section of the ADA (see Chapter 5): essential functions of the job and reasonable accommodations; issues surrounding disclosure; and examples of accommodation strategies and information regarding costs, including the fact that accommodations may cost nothing. Employers, employees with MS, and rehabilitation professionals are featured throughout the 12-minute DVD. Resources are also provided including the National Multiple Sclerosis Society, the Job Accommodation Network (JAN), the state Vocational Rehabilitation program, the United States Business Leadership Network (BLN), and the Employer Assistance and Recruiting Network (EARN), a program funded by the United States Department of Labor Office of Disability Employment Policy. *MS in the Workplace: A Guide for Employers* is available from the National Multiple Sclerosis Society at www.nationalMSsociety.org or by calling 1-800-344-4867.

Home-Based Employment Interventions

Another job-placement and career-reentry strategy for people with MS is home-based employment. Once viewed by vocational rehabilitation professionals as a demeaning concept because it was thought to exclude people with disabilities from working in normative job settings, home-based employment is a burgeoning area of growth in the general labor market. Thanks to the now common practice of telecommuting, the number of Americans who work primarily at home has more than tripled since 1993 (15). Estimates are that as many as 40 percent of all American workers will be working at home for at least part of the time by the year 2010 (15). In the current economy, home-based employment provides what is fast becoming a normative work opportunity for people with disabilities, and people with MS are often excellent candidates for these jobs.

University of Washington Medical Center Program

The University of Washington Medical Center operates a home-based jobs program for people with MS and other neurological disorders (e.g., epilepsy, traumatic brain injury). Fraser (15) noted that interest among people with MS in arranging home-based work opportunities is exceeded only by demand from Seattle-area employers for qualified home-based workers. He reported that people with MS are ideal candidates for home-based employment because they are experienced workers, and because they typically have well-developed social networks outside of the work environment. This means that they are usually not dependent upon work for their primary means of socialization, and that the convenience of working at home frequently outweighs the lack of personal contact with coworkers. Sectors of the economy that Fraser identified as being particularly fertile for home-based employment include computer software and other technologies, finance and investment brokerage, information processing, and insurance.

Job Accommodation Network Small Business and Self-Employment Service

The Job Accommodation Network (JAN) is a free service of the United States Department of Labor Office of Disability Employment Policy (DOL ODEP). West Virginia University administers the Small Business and Self-Employment Service (SBSES) that offers individuals with disabilities information, counseling, guidance, and referrals regarding self-employment and small business. Topics that SBSES staff can address include starting your own business, managing your own business, and dealing with disability issues. Information is available on their website at www.jan.wvu.edu/sbses or by calling 1-800-526-7234 (voice) or 1-877-781-9403 (TTY).

START-UP/USA

START-UP/USA, Self-Employment Technical Assistance, Resources and Training, is a partnership between Virginia Commonwealth University's Rehabilitation Research and Training Center (RRTC) and Griffin-Hammis and Associates, LLC, and is funded by the United States Department of Labor Office of Disability Employment Policy. This project provides technical assistance and offers educational webcasts on entrepreneurship. Resources are provided to individuals with disabilities who are interested in self-employment. Three sub-projects, in Alaska, Florida, and New York, are charged with the generation of data and information to validate systems capacity-building strategies and systems-change models to help increase self-employment opportunities for individuals with disabilities. The information generated through these model programs will be disseminated nationally for replication through technical assistance and support. Information on START-UP/USA can be found at www.start-up-usa.biz/.

Programs Available to People with All Types of Disabilities

The State-Federal Vocational Rehabilitation Program

Within each state, there is an agency that provides comprehensive vocational rehabilitation (VR) services to individuals with disabilities. This agency may have slightly different names in each state and may offer slightly different services, but each one is part of a program that was established by the Rehabilitation Act of 1973 (see Appendix A). The vocational rehabilitation program combines federal and state funds and, although federally mandated, is carried out by individual state agencies. Rumrill and Hennessey (16) wrote that VR services are defined as an eligibility program rather than entitlement program. This means that one must demonstrate eligibility for its services by having a physical or mental impairment that results in a substantial handicap to employment. There must be reasonable expectation that vocational rehabilitation services can help the individual to gain or maintain employment. Many state agencies work under an "Order of Selection" mandate, which means that services are prioritized for individuals with the most significant disabilities.

Services may vary from state to state. Some of the services that may be available include:

- Vocational evaluation and assessment to determine skills, abilities, interests, and the impact of symptoms on employment
- Specialized assessments addressing computer/assistive technology needs
- Vocational guidance and counseling
- Medical appliances and prosthetic devices, if needed, to increase the individual's ability to work
- Vocational training and education
- Occupational tools and equipment
- Job development and placement services
- Follow-along services
- Postemployment services

VR services are available for people who are looking to gain or maintain employment. A person does not have to be unemployed to apply for services from his or her state VR agency. For the individual with MS, one of the challenges may be demonstrating significant enough symptoms under the Order of Selection mandate. With invisible symptoms or symptoms that come and go, demonstrating significant impact may be a challenge. It is important to discuss all the symptoms that a person presently experiences, the symptoms experienced in the past, how the course of the disease changes over time, and the impact symptoms may have in the workplace. In addition, most states also take financial criteria into account when funding services. Many of the specialized assessments and vocational guidance and counseling services, however, can be performed regardless of an individual's financial situation. In some situations, the individual may be expected to contribute financially toward the cost of his or her program, with the state VR agency contributing a portion as well.

Disability and Business Technical Assistance Centers

The Disability and Business Technical Assistance Centers (DBTACs), also known as the ADA and IT Technical Assistance Centers, were established by the National Institute on Disability and Rehabilitation Research (NIDRR) to provide information, training, and technical assistance to employers, people with disabilities, and other entities with responsibilities under the ADA. There are 10 regional centers throughout the United States (see Appendix B). Though the regional centers may vary somewhat in their provisions, all centers provide the following:

- Technical assistance
- Education and training
- Materials dissemination
- Information and referral
- Public awareness
- Local capacity building

Information and assistance is available on issues regarding the various titles or sections of the ADA including employment, public accommodations, public services, and communications. Centers may also be able to address other key legislation including the Family and Medical Leave Act and the Rehabilitation Act of 1973. Local DBTACs can be contacted by calling 1-800-949-4232 (voice/TTY) or online at www.dbtac.vcu.edu.

The Job Accommodation Network

The Job Accommodation Network (JAN) is a free service of the United States Department of Labor Office of Disability Employment Policy (ODEP). JAN's mission is to facilitate the employment and

84

retention of workers with disabilities by providing employers, employment providers, people with disabilities, their family members, and other interested parties with information on job accommodations, self-employment, and small business opportunities. JAN has been providing assistance since 1984. JAN consultants can assist employers to determine appropriate accommodations for employees, gain a better understanding of their responsibilities under the ADA and Rehabilitation Act, and get answers to accessibility questions. For employees and people with disabilities, JAN consultants can help brainstorm accommodation strategies given particular symptoms and job duties, educate individuals about their rights and responsibilities under the ADA and other disability legislation, address the connection between disclosure and the proper way of requesting accommodations, and provide contact information for state government vocational rehabilitation and community agencies. JAN also makes its services available to rehabilitation professionals. JAN can be contacted on-line at www.jan.wvu.edu or by telephone at 1-800-526-7234 (voice) or 1-877-781-9403 (TTY). This free service provides excellent resources and technical assistance in implementing reasonable accommodations in the workplace. Research has demonstrated that the majority of accommodations used by people with MS in the workplace cost little or nothing to implement (1).

Summary

Existing research, clinical reports, and testimonials from people with MS have consistently documented the myriad of difficulties that people with MS encounter as they attempt to seek, secure, and maintain employment following their diagnoses. Indeed, the fact that more than half of these qualified, capable, and productive workers disengage from the work force before reaching retirement age points toward significant gaps in research, program development, and service delivery—gaps that, left unfilled, will continue to deprive society of the vast labor resource that exists within the MS community.

The troubling employment outcomes that currently await people with MS as the disease progresses constitute the bad news, but the good news lies in the numerous programs, services, and interventions that have been developed over the past three decades to promote employment opportunities for Americans with MS. Some of these initiatives are specific to the needs of people with MS, whereas others include people with various types of adult-onset chronic illnesses and still others are available to people with disabilities in general. Taken in aggregate, the MS Employment Assistance Service, Project Alliance, Operation Job Match, the Career Possibilities Project, the Progressive Request Model Intervention, the Job Raising Program, home-based employment programs, Career Crossroads, MS in the Workplace, University of Washington Medical Center, START-UP/USA, the state-federal Vocational Rehabilitation program, the Job Accommodation Network, and the Disability and Business Technical Assistance Centers provide a formidable array of information, technical assistance, advocacy, and direct services that can greatly aid people with MS in continuing their careers after this highly intrusive disease begins to manifest itself.

Generally speaking, people who work are healthier, happier, and have greater access to resources than people who do not work, and paid employment can be an important means of protecting one's assets, maintaining one's sense of identity, staying busy, and maintaining a sense of normalcy and purpose in the face of an unpredictable and interruptive chronic illness like MS. In the endeavor to resume or maintain one's career while coping with MS, the services, programs, and supports described in this chapter can be valuable resources for people with MS, their employers, friends and significant others, rehabilitation professionals, and health care providers.

References

1. Rumrill, P. (2006). Help to stay at work: Vocational rehabilitation strategies for people with multiple sclerosis. *Multiple Sclerosis in Focus, 7*, 14–18.
2. LaRocca, N.G., & Hall, H.L. (1990). Multiple sclerosis program: A model for neuropsychiatric disorders. *New Directions for Mental Health Services, 45*, 49–64.
3. Nissen, S. (2003). *Final report on the Telework Program (unpublished)*. Washington, DC: Operation Job Match/National Multiple Sclerosis Society.
4. Hall, H. (1991). *Final report on the Job Raising Program*. Baltimore: The Development Team.
5. Rumrill, P., Roessler, R., & Cook, B. (1998). Improving career re-entry outcomes for people with multiple sclerosis: A comparison of two approaches. *Journal of Vocational Rehabilitation, 10*(3), 241–252.
6. LaRocca, N.G. (1995). *Employment and multiple sclerosis*. New York: National Multiple Sclerosis Society.
7. Rumrill, P.D., Jr. (1996). *Employment issues and multiple sclerosis*. New York: Demos Vermande.
8. Roessler, R. (1996). The role of assessment in enhancing the vocational potential of people with multiple sclerosis. *Work, 6*, 191–201.
9. Rumrill, P.D., Jr., Roessler, R.T., & Denny, G.S. (1997). Increasing participation in the accommodation request process among employed people with multiple sclerosis: A career maintenance self-efficacy intervention. *Journal of Job Placement, 13*(1), 5–9.

10. Roessler, R., & Rumrill, P.D., Jr. (1995). *Enhancing productivity on your job: The "win-win" approach to reasonable accommodations.* New York: National Multiple Sclerosis Society.
11. Matkin, R. (1995). Private sector rehabilitation. In S. Rubin & R. Roessler (Eds.), *Foundations of the vocational rehabilitation process.* Austin: PRO-ED, pp. 375–398.
12. Rumrill, P. (1993). Increasing the frequency of accommodation requests among employed people with multiple sclerosis. Unpublished Doctoral Dissertation. Fayetteville: University of Arkansas.
13. Sumner, G. (1995). *Project Alliance: A job retention program for employees with chronic illnesses and their employers.* New York: National Multiple Sclerosis Society.
14. Kraft, G., Freal, J., & Coryell, J. (1986). Disability, disease duration, and rehabilitation service needs in multiple sclerosis: Patient perspectives. *Archives of Physical Medicine and Rehabilitation, 67,* 164–168.
15. Fraser, R.T. (1999). Rehabilitation counselor placement-related attributes in the present economy: A project with industry perspective. *Rehabilitation Counseling Bulletin, 42*(4), 343–353.
16. Rumrill, P.D. & Hennessey, M.L. (2007). In R.C. Kalb (Ed.), *Multiple sclerosis: The questions you have, the answers you need.* 3rd Edition. New York: Demos Medical Publishing, pp. 347–376.

Employment and the Americans with Disabilities Act

Mary L. Hennessey

Phillip D. Rumrill, Jr.

I N THIS CHAPTER, we provide an overview of the employment provisions of the Americans with Disabilities Act of 1990 (ADA). The ADA was the first comprehensive legislation passed by any country in the world to prohibit discrimination on the basis of disability. The ADA guarantees full participation in society for people with disabilities in much the same way that the Civil Rights Act of 1964 guarantees the rights of all people regardless of race, gender, national origin, and religion (1). In fact, there were several unsuccessful attempts in the 1960s and 1970s to amend the Civil Rights Act of 1964 to include people with disabilities as a protected class (2). By the 1980s, disability advocates had focused their efforts toward the introduction and ultimate enactment of a stand-alone civil rights law for people with disabilities. Combining some of the intentions and provisions of Section 504 of the Rehabilitation Act and the 1964 Civil Rights Act, the ADA has five titles: Employment, Public Services, Public Accommodations, Communications (telephone systems), and Miscellaneous. The ADA primarily, but not exclusively, applies to protections for "disabled" individuals. Individuals are considered to be "disabled" if they meet at least one of the following criteria: (a) have a physical or mental impairment that substantially limits one or more of their life activities, (b) have a record of such an impairment, or (c) are regarded as having such an impairment (3). Other people are protected by the ADA under certain circumstances including (a) an individual who has an association with a person known to have a disability and (b) those who are coerced or subjected to retaliation for assisting people with disabilities in asserting their rights under the ADA (4).

Title I of the ADA took effect July 26, 1992, and prohibits private employers, state and local governments, employment agencies, and labor unions from discriminating against qualified individuals with disabilities in job application procedures, hiring, firing, advancement, compensation, job training, and other terms, conditions, and privileges of employment. Title II of the ADA addresses public services sponsored or provided by state and local government instrumentalities (including public schools and state colleges and universities), the National Railroad Passenger Corporation, and other commuter authorities. These entities cannot refuse participation in programs and activities to people with disabilities that they offer to nondisabled people. Also included in Title II of the ADA is the accessibility of public transportation systems. Title III covers privately held accommodations that are open to the public such restaurants, hotels, grocery stores, retail stores, and privately owned transportation systems. Under Title III, any new construction and modifications must be accessible to people with disabilities. In existing facilities, barriers to service must be removed if doing so would be readily feasible. Title IV pertains to telecommunications companies. In offering services to the general public, these companies must have telephone relay services available to individuals who use telecommunication devices for the deaf (TTYs) or similar devices. Title V is called miscellaneous, and it includes a provision prohibiting either (a) threatening or coercing or (b) retaliating against a person with a disability or those attempting to assist people with disabilities in asserting their rights under the ADA.

Given the subject of this book, this chapter focuses on Title I of the ADA and the employment protections it provides for people with MS and other disabling conditions. We will define key terms and provisions of Title I, describe the reasonable accommodation process as an important vehicle for job retention, and present remediation and enforcement procedures that the United States Equal Employment Opportunity Commission (EEOC) has established to redress workplace discrimination. The emphasis of this chapter can be best described as "knowledge is power." By understanding the landmark civil rights guarantees provided by the ADA, developing strategies for invoking one's right to nondiscriminatory treatment, and asserting oneself if discrimination does occur the reader will be able to seek, secure, and maintain employment as an informed and confident self-advocate.

Key Terms and Provisions of Title I
Covered Employers
All public and private employers with 15 or more employees must comply with the provisions set forth in Title I of the ADA (3). The federal government, Native American tribes, and tax-exempt private membership clubs are not covered. Religious organizations, labor unions, and businesses that utilize temporary employment services are covered employers under Title I.

Individual with a Disability
As stated previously, the ADA defines an individual with a disability as a person who (a) has a physical or mental impairment which substantially limits functioning in one or more major life activities, (b) has a record of such an impairment, or (c) is regarded as having such an impairment. Major life activities include, but are not limited to, walking, seeing, hearing, speaking, learning, working, concentrating, sleeping, lifting, interacting with others, and self-care (3). When using the term *substantially limits*, the ADA considers either "the inability to perform the major life activity or a significant restriction as to the condition, manner, or duration under which the average person in the general population can perform the same major life activity" (1, p. 91). Rubin and Roessler (1) pointed out that work is a major life activity, and many employees have leveled charges against their employers due to discrimination based on their disabilities in terminating their employment. In fact, as of 2005, more than 4,000 Americans with MS had filed complaints of employment discrimination under the ADA with the United States EEOC (5). As it applies to the major life activity of working, the term *substantially limits* means "significantly restricted in the ability to perform either a class of jobs or a broad range of jobs in various classes as compared to the average person having comparable training, skills and abilities. The inability to perform a single, particular job does not constitute a substantial limitation in the major life activity of work (1, p. 92)." Individuals not protected by Title I of the ADA include (a) people with disabilities who pose a direct threat to the health or safety of themselves or others in the workplace; (b) active abusers of illegal

substances; (c) employees who use alcohol during work; (d) people who are homosexual, transvestites, bisexual, or transsexual (sexual orientation is not considered a disabling condition); (e) voyeurs or people who have other sexual disorders; (f) people who have disorders of kleptomania, compulsive gambling, or pyromania; and (g) people whose medical conditions can be mitigated with assistive technology, medication, or surgery (3).

Qualified Individual with a Disability

Under Title I of the ADA, a qualified person with a disability is one who satisfies the primary requirements of the position and who can perform the fundamental duties (i.e., essential functions) of the job with or without reasonable accommodations. The employer is not required to give preference to applicants with disabilities or to hire or retain an employee with a disability who does not have the required training, skills, and/or experience. The ADA offers no protection for employees whose disabilities have progressed to the point where they are unable to perform the essential functions of their jobs.

Essential Job Functions

Essential job functions are those primary duties which the worker must be capable of performing with reasonable accommodations if required (1). A function is considered essential when (a) the position exists to perform the function; (b) there are a limited number of other employees available to perform the function, or among whom the function can be distributed; and/or (c) the function is highly specialized, and the person in the position is hired for her or his special expertise and ability to perform the function. Essential functions do not include tasks that are marginal or unnecessary to performing the primary duties of the job (such as requiring a driver's license when driving is not required to carry out the work-related tasks, [1]). In ADA Title I court decisions, employers have been given wide latitude in determining what constitutes essential functions of particular jobs. Essential functions must be delineated in a written job description that is given to all applicants and made available to any current employees who request it, but the decision regarding whether a particular function is essential to the job itself has been deferred almost exclusively to the employer (1,6). Essential functions can be identified in a job analysis conducted by a trained rehabilitation professional (7).

Reasonable Accommodations

Reasonable accommodations are modifications to the job or to the work environment that enable qualified people with disabilities to perform the essential functions of their positions. Types of reasonable accommodations include:

- Restructuring of existing facilities
- Restructuring of the job
- Modification of work schedules
- Reassignment to a vacant position
- Modification of equipment
- Installation of new equipment
- Provision of qualified readers and interpreters
- Modification of application and examination procedures or training materials
- Flexible personal leave policies
- Use of supported employment programs

Reasonable accommodations do not include (a) eliminating an essential job function; (b) lowering production standards that are applied to all employees (although an employer may have to provide reasonable accommodations to enable an employee with a disability to meet production standards); (c) providing personal use items such as prosthetic limbs, wheelchairs, eyeglasses, hearing aids, or similar devices, and (d) excusing a violation of uniformly applied conduct rules that are job related and consistent with business necessity (e.g., violence, threats of violence, stealing, destruction of property). Also, as the term *reasonable* implies, an employer is not required to provide an accommodation that constitutes an undue hardship for the business or agency (3).

Undue Hardship

Undue hardship refers to any accommodation that exceeds the bounds of practicality. An accommodation may be considered an undue hardship if it costs more than alternatives that are equally effective, requires extensive or disruptive renovations, or negatively affects other employees and/or customers. Undue hardships are determined on a case-by-case basis using criteria such as the cost and nature of the requested accommodation, the overall financial resources of the facility, and the type of operation of the employer (3).

Reasonable Accommodation Process

For applicants or employees wishing to request a reasonable accommodation in the workplace, Title I regulations (3) prescribe a collaborative, nonadversarial process involving the applicant or employee and the employer. The steps of this process are (8,9):

1. The applicant/employee initiates a request for accommodation (preferably but not necessarily in written form).
2. The applicant/employee and employer collaborate to identify factors that limit the person's ability to perform the job's essential functions.
3. Using the applicant/employee as a resource, the employer identifies a variety of accommodations that would reduce or remove disability-related barriers to job performance.
4. The employer assesses the cost effectiveness of each accommodation strategy to determine which one(s) could be implemented with the least economic hardship.
5. The employer implements an appropriate accommodation, considering the applicant/employee's preferences when two equivalent accommodations have been identified.

Existing research underscores how important reasonable accommodations can be to workers with MS. In a survey of people with MS who had disengaged from the workforce, Duggan et al. (10) reported that only one of five respondents had been provided with on-the-job accommodations. Employed people with MS in Roessler and Rumrill's (11) study reported using a number of on-the-job accommodations to help them maintain their careers. In order of frequency, these strategies included the installation of new equipment (e.g., large-print computer program for a worker with a visual impairment), restructuring of the job (e.g., having a person with tremors in her hands answer phones rather than perform data-entry tasks), modification of work schedules (e.g., allowing the worker to take an extended lunch break during which she could take a nap as a means of combating fatigue), restructuring of existing facilities (e.g., installing a wheelchair-accessible restroom), change in location of the worksite (e.g., home-based employment), reassignment to another position, provision of personal assistance services (e.g., a driver), and modification of equipment. Perhaps most importantly, Roessler and Rumrill (11) noted that more than half of the accommodations identified by respondents had cost their employers nothing at all to implement.

Before becoming eligible for a reasonable accommodation, the workers or applicants must disclose their disability status to their employers and make a request for the accommodation in question. This does not mean, however, that people must disclose their underlying diagnosis or disabling condition. Employers generally do not have the right to know that employees or applicants have MS, only that they have a disability and need an accommodation to perform an essential function of the job they hold or wish to hold (12).

SPECIAL NOTE TO PEOPLE WITH MS REGARDING DISCLOSURE AND THE REASONABLE ACCOMMODATION PROCESS. In general, the best reason for disclosing your disability status is that you foresee a need for a reasonable accommodation on your job. If symptoms of your illness are obvious to others, if they have begun to interfere with your job performance, and/or if you have been receiving feedback from your employer that there are problems with your performance, you may want to approach your employer about possible accommodations. Although you do not have to disclose the underlying cause of your disability (i.e., your MS), it is important to frame your disability status in functional terms: "I am a person with a disability, and I have been having difficulty performing X and Y on my job. I would like to discuss some ways to accommodate these difficulties—some strategies that will enable me to continue being a productive employee."

It is also important to note that you need not reference the ADA specifically in your discussions with your employer. In fact, the National Multiple Sclerosis Society advocates a "win-win" approach to on-the-job accommodations in which the employee with MS keeps his or her legal protections out of the dialog with the employer to every extent possible. The best rationale for reasonable accommodations is that they will help you to maintain or enhance your productivity on the job. This benefits both you and the employer, and it demonstrates your willingness to engage in a cooperative, nonadversarial process of identifying and implementing cost-effective accommodations. This approach is almost always more effective than invoking your civil rights in a formal way, or threatening to sue your employer if he or she does not meet your needs. The best advice about disclosure and the accommodation request process is to:

● Be direct but friendly.
● Frame your disability-related work limitations in functional terms.

- Focus on your accommodation needs rather than your medical diagnosis.
- Emphasize the mutual benefits of providing you with on-the-job accommodations.
- Use your legal rights and recourses under the ADA if, and only if, your employer refuses to provide an appropriate accommodation to meet your stated needs.

Beyond Reasonable Accommodations: Other ADA Title I Requirements

Although reasonable accommodations are an important part of the ADA, the employment protections available to people with disabilities go far beyond on-the-job accommodations. Under Title I, people with disabilities have the civil right to enjoy the same benefits and privileges of employment as their nondisabled coworkers and to have personnel decisions made without regard to disability status. Workers may not be harassed on the basis of their disabilities, and the compensation they receive must be commensurate with their qualifications and productivity irrespective of disability (3).

The *Technical Assistance Manual* developed by the EEOC is available to assist employers (i.e., private, state, and local governments), other covered entities (i.e., employment agencies, labor unions, joint labor-management committees), and those with disabilities to learn about their rights and obligations under Title I. The Manual offers guidance on the application of legal requirements established in the statute and the EEOC's regulations. In addition, it provides resources for references to aid in compliance on the part of employers and employees with disabilities. This Manual is updated with supplements on a periodic basis.

The Manual is divided into two parts. Part One explains legal requirements in practical terms including: who is protected by and those required to comply with the ADA; permissions and prohibitions of the law with respect to creating qualification standards, evaluating the qualifications and capacities of people with disabilities to perform particular jobs, and requiring medical examinations; the nature of the obligation to make a reasonable accommodation; how the law's non-discrimination provisions apply to aspects of the employment process including promotion, transfer, termination, compensation, leave, fringe benefits, and contractual arrangements; and how ADA provisions and requirements affect legal obligations and policies related to drug, alcohol, and workers' compensation practices and policies. The second part of the Manual is a directory that lists public and private organizations and agencies that offer information, expertise, and technical assistance on aspects of employing people with disabilities, including reasonable accommodations.

Areas of employment in which employers may not discriminate against people with disabilities include application, promotion, testing, medical examinations, hiring, layoff/recall, assignments, termination, evaluation, compensation, disciplinary actions, leave, training, and benefits. Specific actions that the ADA considers discriminatory include (a) limiting, segregating, or classifying a job applicant or employee in a way that adversely affects employment opportunities because of his or her disability; (b) participating in contractual or other arrangements or relationships that subjects an employer's qualified applicant or employee with a disability to discrimination; (c) denying employment opportunities to a qualified individual because he or she has a relationship or association with a person with a disability; (d) refusing to make reasonable accommodations to the known physical or mental limitations of a qualified applicant or employee with a disability unless the accommodation would pose an undue hardship on the business; (e) using qualification standards, employment tests, or other selection criteria that screen out or tend to screen out an individual with a disability unless they are job related and necessary for the business; (f) failing to use employment tests in the most effective manner to measure actual abilities; and (g) discriminating against an individual because he or she has opposed an employment practice of the employer or filed a complaint, testified, assisted or participated in an investigation, proceeding, or hearing to enforce provisions of the Act.

Hiring, Recruitment, Applications, Preemployment Inquiries, and Testing

An employer must follow nondiscrimination requirements when recruiting applicants for a job and during the application process itself. An individual with a disability has the same right to participate in the application process and be considered for the advertised job as do all other people. The employer does not have the right to ask any preemployment questions regarding the applicant's disability status, but the employer may ask questions related to the applicant's ability to perform specific job functions. The employer may also ask the applicant with a disability to explain or demonstrate how he or she would perform these functions. The employer can make a job offer conditional on the results of a post-offer medical examination but only if all applicants are subject to such a condition. Tests for illegal drugs are not considered part of a medical examination and may be required of the applicant at any time. Any testing performed must be job related and consistent with the necessity of the position or business of the employer. Testing cannot be used to screen out persons on the basis of their disability. Tests must also measure the skills and aptitudes of the individual rather than the impaired sensory, intellectual, physical, or speaking skills unless those are job-related skills that the test is designed to measure.

The EEOC's *Technical Assistance Manual* suggests that employers include information regarding essential job functions in all job announcements, advertisements, and other recruitment notices as a means of attracting the most qualified applicants, both with disabilities and without. Employers can also indicate directly on the announcement that they do not discriminate on the basis of disability or any other legally prohibited basis. As far as the format of the announcement is concerned, employers do not have to provide written information in alternative formats in advance, but should make accessible formats available upon request.

As an example, job information should be available in a location that is accessible to people with MS who have mobility impairments. If a job advertisement provides only a telephone number to call for information, a telecommunication device for the deaf (TDD) number should be included unless a telephone relay service has been established. Printed job information in an employment office or on employee bulletin boards should be made available, as needed, to persons with MS who have visual or other reading impairments. Preparing information in large print will help make it available to some people with visual impairments and large print can make postings "stand out" to all interested parties on bulletin boards or in newspaper advertisements. Information can be recorded on a cassette or read to applicants with more severe vision impairments and those who have other disabilities that limit reading ability.

The ADA does not require employers to implement special activities to recruit individuals with disabilities. Recruitment activities that have the effect of screening out probable applicants with disabilities may violate the statute. Employers are encouraged to expand their recruitment programs to attract the most diverse set of qualified applicants. For example, if an employer conducts a recruitment activity at a college campus, job fair, or other location that is physically inaccessible, or does not make its recruitment activity accessible at such locations to people with visual, hearing, or other disabilities, that employer may be liable if a charge of discrimination is filed.

As stated previously, an employer may not make any preemployment inquiries regarding a person's disability status. This protection may be particularly important for a person with a hidden disability which is often the case for people with MS. An employer can still obtain the necessary information regarding an applicant's qualifications, including medical information that pertains to assessing the applicant's qualifications and gives assurances that his or her health and safety are maintained during employment. The ADA requires that these inquiries are made at two different stages in the hiring process. Before a job offer is made, an employer can ask questions about an applicant's ability to perform specific functions of the job, may not ask about a disability, and may make a job offer that is conditioned on acceptable results of a postoffer medical examination. After the employer makes a conditional job offer and before the person begins to work, the employer may request that the applicant answer health-related questions or participate in a medical examination. This is only the case if the employer requires all applicants (postoffer) to have a medical examination or answer health-related questions.

The employer is not permitted to ask any disability-related questions on a job application. Some examples of the questions that may not be asked are: Have you ever been hospitalized? If so, for what condition? Have you ever been treated for any mental condition? Have you had a major illness in the last 5 years? Is there any health-related reason you may not be able to perform the job for which you are applying? These are just a few of the types of questions that an employer is not permitted to ask on an application form. Information that an employer is permitted to ask on application forms or in interviews must be related to determining if an applicant can perform specific job functions. The questions must focus on the applicant's abilities, not on a disability. For example, an employer may provide the applicant with a job description or a list of specific job functions with the application, or the employer may describe the functions of the job. At this point, the employer then may ask whether the applicant can perform these functions. The applicant could be asked if he or she is able to perform the tasks listed with or without accommodations. If the applicant indicates that he or she can perform the job with accommodations, the employer may then ask how he would complete the tasks and what accommodations would be needed. An application can also state that the applicant can request accommodations to partici-pate in the application/interview process. This may include assistance in filling out the application form or accommodations if testing is required.

The interview process includes the same considerations as the job application process. An employer may not ask a person about his or her disability, but can ask about the applicant's ability to perform the essential functions of the job being interviewed for and about any needed accommodations. If an applicant has a visible disability (e.g., uses a wheelchair, has a guide dog, uses a cane), or has provided the employer with information about his or her disability, the interviewer is still not permitted to ask questions about the nature of the applicant's disability, the severity of the applicant's disability, the condition causing the dis-ability, prognosis or expectation regarding the disability, or whether the interviewee will need extended leave or special treatment related to the disability. The interviewer can provide specific information related to the job functions and ask whether the interviewee can perform those tasks with or without an accommodation.

For example, the interviewer would explain that the position as a mailroom clerk is responsible for accepting incoming mail and packages, sorting those items, and transporting the items in a cart to various offices in two buildings. The clerk will also have to accept packages that weigh up to 50 pounds and place them on storage shelves that are as high as 6 feet. The interviewer could then ask the interviewee if he or she could perform those specific tasks and if he or she could perform them with or without a reasonable accommodation.

Note that the interviewer may also ask about the individual's ability to perform all functions of a job, not just the essential functions. For example, a job description for a clerical position includes the following functions: (a) transcribing dictation and drafts of written reports into final documents for other staff, (b) proofreading documents, (c) creating and maintaining files, (d) scheduling and arranging meetings and confer-ences, (e) logging documents and correspondence, (f) using the telephone, (g) distributing documents to staff, (h) copying documents using the copy machine, and (i) intermittent travel to conferences to perform clerical tasks. Functions a through f are considered to be essential functions of the job, while g through i are marginal tasks. The interviewer can ask the applicant about his or her ability to perform all nine functions; suppose that the applicant had mobility problems resulting from MS and could not perform functions g through i. This applicant should not be screened out of candidacy for this position because functions g through i are not essential elements of the clerical or secretarial position. The applicant should be evaluated on the ability to perform six essential functions, with or without an accommodation.

An applicant has the right to equal access in the interview process. Therefore, an employer must provide an accommodation if needed by the applicant. As indicated earlier, the employer should note this on the application. Needed accommodations for the interview may include a reader for a person with a visual impairment, an accessible location for a person who uses a wheelchair, or an interpreter for a person who is deaf.

Employers are permitted to conduct background and reference checks on applicants with and without disabilities. They may not obtain this information prior to making a conditional job offer. The employer may not ask for any information regarding the applicant from a previous employer, family member, or other source that was not requested from the applicant himself or herself. Before making a conditional job offer, an employer may not ask previous employers or other sources about an applicant's disability, illness, workers' compensation history, or any other questions that the employer itself is not permitted to ask of the applicant. In a reference or background check, the employer may ask the applicant's previous employer about the applicant's job performance, the quantity and quality of the applicant's work, how job functions were performed, record of attendance, and other job-related issues that do not relate to disability. If the applicant has indicated his or her disability status and that he or she could perform the job with a reasonable accommodation, the employer may ask the previous employer about accommodations made in the past.

Many types of tests may be used by employers to determine if an applicant is qualified to perform a particular job. The ADA has two primary requirements in regard to testing: (a) the test must be job related and consistent with business necessity if the test screens out or tends to screen out a person with a disability or a class of individuals on the basis of disability, and (b) the applicant must have access to reasonable accommodations if necessary. The requirement regarding testing applies to all types of tests including, but not limited to, aptitude, agility, and intelligence tests; tests of skills and knowledge; and job demonstrations. A test will be an accurate predictor of job performance of any job applicant when it directly or closely measures actual skills and abilities needed to do the job. A keyboarding test, sales demonstration test, or other type of job performance test would provide information regarding an applicant's actual ability to perform the job as opposed to a test that measures general qualities thought to be desirable in a job. If a person with a disability is screened out for a reason unrelated to the disability, the ADA does not apply. Even if the test is job related and justified as a necessity, the employer is obligated to provide an accommodation if the applicant is in need of one.

If a person has impaired sensory, speaking, or manual skills, the ADA requires that the test be given in a format or manner that does not require use of the impaired skill unless the test is designed to measure that skill. This requirement ensures that a person's job skills, aptitudes, or other measures being tested are accurately reflected rather than the person's impaired skills. This requirement allows people with disabilities the equal opportunity to apply for and demonstrate appropriate job skills along with all other qualified applicants. Recall, the employer is not required to provide an alternative testing format for any person with an impaired skill if the purpose of the test is to measure that skill. For example, providing extra time for test taking may be a reasonable accommodation for a person with MS who is experiencing visual difficulties, cognitive impairment, or fine motor disturbances. Results of a timed test should not be used to exclude an applicant with a disability unless the skill of speed is an essential component of the job for which the applicant is applying.

The employer is required to provide an accommodation if he or she is aware of the need for that accommodation or has received a request. Generally, it is the responsibility of the applicant to request any accommodations needed for testing. The employer may require that the applicant request a specific accommodation within a particular time frame before the test is given and also require documentation of the need for the accommodation. There are circumstances when an individual with a disability may not think he or she will need an accommodation for a particular test. For example, an applicant knows that there will be a reading test required for the job he or she is applying for. The applicant has a visual impairment and has specially designed glasses to accommodate his or her need for reading printed material. When the test is given, the applicant discovers that the glasses are not adequate because of the variation in contrast from high to low color between the ink and the paper that the test is printed on. In this situation, the applicant may request an accommodation at that point in time and the employer would be required to provide the accommodation, such as providing an alternate format of the test or rescheduling the test as long as it would not impose an undue hardship on the employer. The employer is not required to provide the specific accommodation that the applicant requests but he or she must provide an effective accommodation. Examples of alternative test formats and accommodations include: (a) giving a written test instead of an oral test for a person with a speech impairment or difficulty hearing; (b) providing a test in large print or Braille for a person with a visual impairment; (c) permitting the use of a tape recorder, dictation, or computer for recording answers if the person has limited use of his or her hands or a visual or learning disability; (d) offering extra time for test taking if the person has a learning disability or impaired writing abilities; (e) including scheduled breaks during the testing process for a person with chronic fatigue; (f) providing a separate room for testing for a person who may be easily distracted; and (g) using other means of evaluation such as interview, work experience, education, certifications, or job demonstration for a trial period.

Medical Examinations

There are several steps to note regarding the order of job offer and requirements for medical examinations. Before an applicant is offered a job and before that applicant is hired by an employer, the employer may not require the applicant to participate in a medical examination, or respond to any questions that is asked about medical history or workers' compensation claims. This is necessary because some employers rely on medical policies or physician assessments that overestimate the impact of a particular condition on an individual or underestimate the ability of an individual to manage his or her condition. Medical policies of a company that focus on disability as opposed to ability of its workers are discriminatory under the ADA (13).

When an applicant has been offered the position but has not yet begun employment, the employer may make the offer conditional on the results of a preemployment medical examination—provided that all applicants are required to participate in the postoffer, preemployment examination. An employer may not require an applicant who disclosed his or her MS during the job interview to submit to a preemployment medical examination if such an examination is not standard procedure for all hirees. The sole purpose of the exam is to determine if a person has the physical or mental qualifications necessary to perform the job being offered. For example, if a construction job requires continuous heavy physical exertion, a medical examination could be used to determine whether a person with MS could meet the heavy exertion requirement for that position. An applicant may also be questioned at this time regarding previous injuries and history of workers' compensation claims. A postoffer medical examination does not have to be required of all entering employees in all jobs, only to those in the same job category.

If an offer of employment is rescinded following a medical examination, the employer is required to show that the reason(s) for not hiring the individual with the disability were job related and necessary for the business. The employer is also required to show that no reasonable accommodation was possible to enable the individual with the disability to perform the essential functions of the job, or that an accommodation would impose an undue hardship. According to the EEOC, the postoffer medical inquiry or examination cannot preclude an individual with a disability who is currently capable of performing the essential job functions because of assumptions that the disability may cause future injury.

Once the person has been employed, the employer may require a medical examination when there is evidence of safety issues or job performance problems. The employer may also require a medical examination if the examination is required by other federal laws or to determine "fitness" to perform in a different position (13).

A quick note about confidentiality: an employer is required to keep all information regarding medical examinations and inquires in a separate file from the employee's other employment records. The medical record must be marked as confidential, and it is only available under limited conditions specified by the ADA. The employer should designate only a specific person(s) to have access to the medical files.

Under the ADA, information about the applicant's/employee's medical documentation, or whether the person is a "direct threat" to health and safety may be obtained from sources other than a medical doctor. This information may also be provided by rehabilitation experts, occupational or physical therapists, psychologists, and any other persons knowledgeable regarding the individual with the disability.

For authoritative information regarding medical examinations, consult the EEOC's *Technical Assistance Manual: Title I of the ADA* (13). When an individual is rejected for a job position because of direct threat to health and safety, the employer must demonstrate a significant current risk of substantial harm; the specific risk must be described; the risk must be recorded by objective medical or factual evidence regarding the particular individual; and the employer must determine whether the harm can be eliminated or reduced below the level of direct threat via reasonable accommodation.

The following are examples of postoffer decisions that might be job related and justified by business necessity, and/or where no reasonable accommodation was possible (13, p. 107):

- A person's medical history reveals that the individual sustained serious multiple reinjuries to his back while doing similar work, which have progressively worsened the back condition. Employing this person in this job would incur great risk that he would further reinjure himself.
- The individual's workers' compensation history attests to multiple claims in recent years which have been denied. An employer might have a legitimate business reason to believe that the person has submitted fraudulent claims. Withdrawing a job offer for this reason would not violate the ADA because the decision is not based on disability.
- A medical examination discloses a diagnosis (such as MS) that would require the individual's frequent lengthy absence from work for medical treatment, and the job requires daily availability for the next 3 months. In this situation, the individual is not available to execute the essential functions of the job, and no accommodation is possible.

Examples of discriminatory use of examination results that are not job related and justified by business necessity include (13, p. 108):

- A landscaping company sent an applicant for a laborer's job (who had been doing this kind of work for 20 years) for a physical exam. An x-ray revealed that he had a curvature of the spine. The doctor advised the firm not to hire him because there was a risk that he might injure his back at some time in the future. The doctor provided no specific medical documentation that this would happen or was likely to happen. The company provided no description of the job to the doctor. The job actually involved riding a mechanical mower. This unlawful exclusion was based on speculation about future risk of injury, and was not job related.

● An applicant with MS is rejected from a job because the individual cannot lift more than 50 pounds. The job requires lifting such a weight only occasionally. The employer has not considered possible accommodations, such as sharing the occasional heavy weight lifting with another employee or providing a device to assist in lifting.

Nondiscrimination in Other Employment Areas

The areas of hiring, applications, medical examinations, and selection standards provide a major portion of the protections set forth in Title I of the ADA as noted in the above sections. There are several other areas of requirement that are applicable to certain employment activities and practices. To this point in the chapter, it is well established that:

● An employer may not discriminate against a qualified individual with a disability because of the disability, in any employment practice, or any term, condition, or benefit of employment.
● An employer may not deny an employment opportunity because an individual, with or without a disability, has a relationship or association with an individual who has a disability.
● An employer may not participate in a contractual or other arrangement that subjects the employer's qualified applicant or employee with a disability to discrimination.
● An employer may not discriminate or retaliate against any individual, whether or not the individual is disabled, because the individual has opposed a discriminatory practice, filed a discrimination charge, or participated in any way in enforcing the ADA (13).

Specifically, the ADA prohibits discrimination against any individual with a disability who is qualified in the following employment areas: (a) recruitment, advertising, and application procedures; (b) hiring, job upgrade, promotion, tenure, demotion, transfer, layoff, termination, right of return from layoff, and rehiring; (c) scales of pay or any other form of compensation, and changes in compensation; (d) job assignments, job classifications, organizational structures, position descriptions, lines of progression, and seniority lists; (e) leaves of absence, sick leave, or any other leave; (f) fringe benefits available by virtue of employment, whether or not administered by the covered entity; (g) selection and financial support for training, including apprenticeships, professional meetings, conferences, and other related activities, and selection for leaves of absence to pursue training; (h) activities sponsored by a covered entity, including social and recreational programs; and (i) any other term, condition, or privilege of employment (13).

As applied to all employment practices, nondiscrimination means that people with disabilities should have equal access to any and all employment opportunities just as their nondisabled peers. People with MS or another disabling condition should expect that decisions made regarding employment are based on facts and not on assumptions or stereotypes about their disability. Their qualifications are based on their ability to perform all of the essential functions of the job with or without reasonable accommodations, and they may not be precluded from the job because their disability prevents performance of the marginal job functions. Reasonable accommodations must be provided so an individual with a disability may participate in every aspect of employment, unless the accommodation would impose an undue hardship to the employer. Employment practices and policies cannot be used to screen out individuals with disabilities or a class of individuals with disabilities unless the practice is job related and is necessary to the business and in which undue hardship would be caused by the implementation of a reasonable accommodation. An individual with a disability cannot be segregated, classified, or limited by the employer in any way in terms of advancement or job opportunities. A person with a disability should not be in any way treated differently from anyone else in any aspect of employment. This may only occur if a reasonable accommodation is needed or the federal law requires different treatment.

That summary of ADA Title I protections in mind, people with disabilities are also protected in the area of advancement and promotion. Employers should not assume that individuals with a disability are not qualified or not interested in a promotion because of their disability. Employers cannot rule against promotion for people with a disability because they do not want to implement a reasonable accommodation unless it would cause an undue hardship. Employees with a disability should follow the same lines and rules for promotion and should not be put into a separate or special category. All members of management should be aware of the ADA regulations regarding promotion and advancement.

All employees, both disabled and nondisabled, also have the right to access and participate in all training opportunities that lead to advancement and improved job performance. As with promotion, a training opportunity cannot be denied to an individual with a disability because the employer does not want to make a reasonable accommodation for the training to take place (unless it would cause an undue hardship). Accommodations for training are much like any other accommodations that an employee may need to perform his or her job: accessible location; interpreters and notetakers; materials provided in accessible formats, such as large print, Braille, captions; good lighting and ventilation; clarification of concepts; and the opportunity for individualized instruction. It is the employer's responsibility to make sure that accommodations are in place even if an agency is contracted to perform the training.

Workers with disabilities must also enjoy equality in the areas of evaluation, discipline, and discharge. An employer can hold an employee with a disability to the same standards of production and performance as others in similar positions performing essential functions with or without reasonable accommodations. By the same token, an employer can require the employee with a disability to meet the same standards in evaluations related to marginal job functions unless the disability affects the ability to perform the marginal functions. If that is the case, a reasonable accommodation must be implemented unless it would constitute an undue hardship. In the evaluation process, the employer must not consider the employee's disability status and need for the reasonable accommodation—the employer must evaluate the performance based on the outcome with the reasonable accommodation in place. Overall, an employer should not give special considerations when evaluating or disciplining an individual with a disability. The standard cannot be lowered as this is not considered equal employment opportunity. If an employee with a disability is not performing well, the employer can request a medical examination or other professional assessments that are job related to assist the employee in identifying reasonable accommodations that could be implemented. An employer may not terminate an employee with a disability if he or she has refused to provide an accommodation and the reason for the poor performance was a result of the lack of the accommodation.

Regarding equal pay, an employer cannot reduce the pay of an employee with a disability if some of his or her marginal job tasks are eliminated or because specialized equipment is needed as a reasonable accommodation. However, an employee who is reassigned to a lower paying job or who is relegated to part-time employment as an accommodation may be paid a lower compensation amount commensurate with the position and company policies.

The nondiscrimination requirements also apply to any social or recreational activities carried out or provided by the employer, and transportation opportunities offered, and all other benefits and privileges of employment. Employees with disabilities can expect to participate equally in company picnics, parties, shows, ceremonies, or any other social functions through the use of accommodations such as accessible spaces, interpreters, and accessible materials. Break rooms, lounges, cafeterias, and other nonwork facilities must be usable by both disabled and nondisabled employees. Accessibility also applies to exercise rooms, gyms, or health clubs. An employer does not have to eliminate facilities provided to employees because a person with a disability is not able to use certain types of equipment or amenities because of his or her disability.

Enforcement

In the event that a person experiences any of the discriminatory actions prohibited by the ADA that have been discussed to this point in the chapter, there are a number of steps that can be taken to redress unfair treatment in the workplace. Title I of the ADA is enforced by United States Equal Employment Opportunities Commission under the same procedures used to enforce Title VII of the Civil Rights Act of 1964.

Any employee or job applicant may file a charge with the EEOC if he or she believes that discrimination has occurred on the basis of disability. An individual, group, or organization also can file a charge on behalf of another person. The individual or group filing the charge is called the "charging party."

To file a complaint, the charging party should contact the nearest EEOC office (see www.eeoc.gov). If there is no EEOC office nearby, call toll free 1-800-669-4000 (voice) or 1-800-800-3302 (TDD). Readers should not delay in filing charges; the charge must be filed within 180 days of the alleged discriminatory action. If there is a state or local fair employment practices agency that enforces another law prohibiting the same alleged discriminatory practice, it is possible that charges may be filed with the EEOC up to 300 days after the alleged discriminatory act. Even though the charging party has at least 180 days and possibly 300 days to file the complaint following the alleged act of discrimination, we recommend that people with MS file a charge with the EEOC as soon as they have experienced the discriminatory treatment and decided that they wish to make a formal complaint. It is much easier to document discrimination when it is fresh in one's mind. ADA Title I charges can be filed in person, via telephone, or by mail.

Upon receipt of the charge, the EEOC conducts an investigation to determine the likelihood that discrimination occurred. Information that is routinely collected from the charging party during this investigation includes (a) the charging party's name, address, and telephone number (if a charge is filed on behalf of another individual, his or her identity may be kept confidential, unless required for a court action); (b) the employer's name, address, telephone number, and number of employees; (c) the basis or bases of the discrimination claimed by the individual (e.g., disability, race, color, religion, sex, national origin, age, retaliation); (d) the issue or issues involved in the alleged discriminatory act(s) (e.g., hiring, promotion, wages, terms and conditions of employment, discharge); (e) identification of the charging party's alleged disability (e.g., the physical or mental impairment and how it affects major life activities, the record of disability the employer relied upon, or how the employer regarded the individual as disabled); (f) the date of the alleged discriminatory act(s); (g) details of what allegedly happened; and (h) identity of witnesses who have knowledge of the alleged discriminatory acts (13). The person with a disability making the charge may also include additional written or verbatim evidence on his or her behalf. The EEOC has work-sharing agreements with many state and local fair employment agencies, therefore depending on the agreement, some charges may be sent to a state or local agency for investigation; others may be investigated directly by the EEOC.

A person with a disability may file a charge of discrimination on more than one basis. For example, an African American woman with MS who works as an engineer may claim that she was discriminated against by an employer based on her race, her gender, and/or her disability. This hypothetical charging party could file a single charge claiming all three bases or she could file a separate charge for each basis. The individual with a disability may also file a lawsuit against an employer, but he or she must first file the charge with the EEOC. The charging party should request a "right to sue" letter from the EEOC 180 days after the charge was first filed with the local EEOC office. The charging party then has 90 days to file suit after receiving the notice of right to sue. If the suit is filed, the EEOC will usually dismiss the original charges filed with the Commission. "Right to sue" letters are also issued when the EEOC does not believe discrimination occurred or when conciliation attempts fail and the EEOC decides not to sue on the charging party's behalf.

A person with a disability may hesitate to file a claim with the EEOC for fear of retaliation. It is unlawful for an employer or other covered entity to retaliate against someone who files a charge of discrimination, participates in an investigation, or opposes discriminatory practices. If a person filing a charge believes that he or she has been the subject of retaliation, the EEOC should be contacted immediately. Even if an individual has already filed a charge of discrimination, he or she can then file a new charge based on retaliation.

A person may bring a charge against a private employer, state or local government, employment agency, labor union, or joint labor management committee. The "respondent" is the party against whom the charge is filed. Within 10 days after receipt of a charge, the EEOC sends written notification to the respondent and the charging party. The EEOC then begins its investigation by reviewing information received from the charging party and requesting information from the respondent. Information requested from the respondent may include (a) specific information regarding the issues raised in the charge; (b) any witnesses who can provide evidence about issues in the charge; (c) information about the operation of the business, employment process, and workplace; and (d) personnel and payroll records. The charge may be dismissed during the course of the investigation for a variety of reasons. For example, the EEOC may find that the respondent is not covered by the ADA, or that the charge was not filed in a timely manner.

The charging party and respondent will be informed of the preliminary findings of the investigation. Both parties will be provided an opportunity to submit further information. After reviewing all information, the EEOC sends an official "Letter of Determination" to the charging party and the respondent, stating whether it has or has not found "reasonable cause" to believe that discrimination occurred (13). If the inquiry reveals there is no cause to believe discrimination occurred, the EEOC will take no further action. They will issue a "right to sue" letter to the charging party. The party may then initiate a private suit. If the EEOC has found cause for discrimination it will attempt to resolve the issue through conciliation and to obtain full relief consistent with the EEOC's standards for remedies for the charging party (13).

At all stages, the EEOC attempts to resolve a charge without a costly lawsuit. If the EEOC has found cause to believe that discrimination occurred, but cannot resolve the issue through conciliation, the case will be considered for litigation. If the EEOC decides to litigate, a lawsuit will be filed in Federal District Court. If the EEOC decides not to litigate, it will issue a "right-to-sue" as previously described.

Remedies

Remedies or "relief" provided for discrimination in employment may include hiring, reinstatement, promotion, back pay, front pay, reasonable accommodation, or other procedures that will make the individual "whole" (in the condition he or she would have been in if he or she would not have experienced discrimination). Remedies can also include fees such as those incurred from the retention of attorneys, expert witnesses, and court costs. If it is found that intentional discrimination has occurred, the employee may receive compensatory and punitive damages. Categories of damages can include compensation for actual monetary losses, future monetary losses, and mental anguish and inconvenience. Punitive damages may be awarded if an employer functioned in a malicious or reckless manner. There are limits to the amount of damages for future monetary loss and emotional injury that a person may receive. The following are based on the size of the employer (13):

15 to 100 employees—$50,000
101 to 200 employees—$100,000
201 to 500 employees—$200,000
500 or more employees—$300,000

State and local governments are not subject to punitive damages under Title I of the ADA. If cases concern reasonable accommodations, damages (punitive or compensatory) may not be awarded to the charging party if the employer is able to exhibit that a "good faith" effort was made to provide the requested reasonable accommodation.

Summary

With the noble but so far unrealistic aspiration of eliminating discrimination on the basis of disability in all aspects of society, the Americans with Disabilities Act stands as the most important civil rights legislation for people with disabilities in the history of the world. First and foremost among the areas of social activity covered by the ADA is employment. Title I of the ADA provides people with MS and other disabling conditions the civil right to fair treatment in the workplace, and it mandates that all employment and personnel decisions made by covered employers be made without regard to disability. Title I of the ADA also requires covered employers to provide reasonable accommodations to qualified applicants or employees with disabilities, and research indicates that many of the workplace accommodations utilized by Americans with MS cost nothing or very little to implement. Other protections available to people with MS and other disabilities concern hiring, promotion, layoff, sick and vacation leave, firing and termination, medical examinations, employee screening and testing, harassment, intimidation, accessibility of the work setting, and health insurance and other benefits.

For people who encounter workplace discrimination and wish to file a complaint under Title I of the ADA, the first step is to contact the United States Equal Employment Opportunity Commission (www.eeoc.gov). The EEOC investigates the claim, makes a determination as to whether discrimination actually occurred, resolves the issue with the employer if possible, and remands the claim to Federal Circuit Court if the matter cannot be resolved without litigation. Remedies under Title I include hiring or reinstatement, punitive and compensatory damages, back pay, front pay, and court orders to stop discriminatory practices.

By understanding the provisions of Title I of the ADA, people with MS, rehabilitation professionals, and disability advocates can remove or reduce many of the barriers to employment and career development that have plagued the MS community for many years. One major step toward improving the rate of labor force participation among people with MS lies in making sure that the American workplace operates fairly, equitably, and inclusively for all workers. We have come a long way since the ADA was signed into law in 1990, but there remains a long way to go. Knowledge is power, and knowing one's civil rights as a worker and how to address and redress on-the-job discrimination is an important career maintenance strategy in today's diversified and highly competitive global marketplace.

References

1. Rubin, S., & Roessler, R. (2001). *Foundations of the vocational rehabilitation process*. Austin: PRO-ED.
2. Dinerstein, R. (2004). The Americans with Disabilities Act of 1990. *Human Rights: Journal of the Section of Individual Rights & Responsibilities, 31*(3), 10–12.
3. Equal Employment Opportunity Commission, www.eeoc.gov. Retrieved May 20, 2007.

4. Job Accommodation Network, www.jan.wvu.edu. Retrieved June 1, 2007.

5. Rumrill, P. (2006). Help to stay at work: Vocational rehabilitation strategies for people with multiple sclerosis. *Multiple Sclerosis in Focus, 7,* 14–18.

6. Rumrill, P., & Hennessey, M. (Eds.) (2001). *Multiple sclerosis: A guide for rehabilitation and health care professionals.* Springfield, IL: Charles C. Thomas.

7. Dunn, P. (2001). Issues and trends in proprietary rehabilitation. In P. Rumrill, J. Bellini, & L. Koch (Eds.), *Emerging issues in rehabilitation counseling: Perspectives on the new millennium.* Springfield, IL: Charles C. Thomas, pp.173–191.

8. Feldblum, C. (1991). Employment protections. In J. West (Ed.), *The Americans with Disabilities Act: From policy to practice.* New York: Milbank Memorial Fund, pp. 81–110.

9. Rumrill, P.D., Jr. (1996). *Employment issues and multiple sclerosis.* New York: Demos Vermande.

10. Duggan, E., Fagan, P., & Yateman, S. (1993). *Employment factors among individuals with multiple sclerosis.* Unpublished manuscript. New York: National Multiple Sclerosis Society.

11. Roessler, R.T., & Rumrill, P.D., Jr. (1995). The Work Experience Survey: A structured interview approach to worksite accommodation planning. *Journal of Job Placement and Development, 11*(1), 15–19.

12. Rumrill, P., & Hennessey, M. (2004). Key employment concerns for people with multiple sclerosis. In R. Kalb (Ed.), *Multiple sclerosis: The questions you have, the answers you need.* 3rd Edition. New York: Demos Medical Publishing, pp. 347–376.

13. Job Accommodation Network (2007). *Technical Assistance Manual: Title I of the ADA,* www.jan.wvu.edu/links/ADAtam1, Retrieved May 29, 2007.

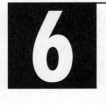

Federal Laws Concerning Continuation of Benefits, Health Insurance Portability, and Family and Medical Leave

Kimberly Calder

U NLIKE VIRTUALLY EVERY OTHER industrialized nation in the world today, the United States does not guarantee access to health care as a right of citizenship. Instead, the United States has historically relied on employers and trade unions to provide health insurance to workers and their dependents as a benefit of employment or membership (1,2). And while many in America today, including many people with multiple sclerosis (MS), get some or all of their health insurance from Medicare, Medicaid, the Veterans' Administration, or other government sources, this chapter focuses on employer-based health insurance and the rights and responsibilities of those who benefit from it. The chapter also describes the provisions of the Family and Medical Leave Act, which provides Americans with MS or other serious health conditions and their immediate family members the right to unpaid leave while protecting their jobs and employee benefits.

Over the past 20 years, Congress has passed legislation to help prevent workers and their dependents from becoming uninsured and suffering financial loss from illness or disability. As such, these laws provide a framework of worker protections within our employer-based health insurance system, with state laws and government programs filling in many of the gaps. Because helping people with MS to maintain health insurance and access health care without interruption is an important

115

goal for everyone in the MS community, staying insured is an essential consideration in examining the employment issues facing people with MS.

A basic knowledge of employee rights and protections, as well as the deadlines and requirements that must be met to access these protections, is critical to good planning and uninterrupted coverage. Often referred to by their acronyms, COBRA (Consolidated Omnibus Reconciliation Act), HIPAA (Health Insurance Portability and Accountability Act), and FMLA (Family and Medical Leave Act), this chapter summarizes these three federal laws and highlights their various and occasionally overlapping provisions. From examples, readers will see how these laws coordinate to address the individual and common needs of people living with MS. And while there is no denying the complexity of some of their provisions, the most important things to know about any of these statutes is, first, that they exist and, second, where to get specific information to help tailor them to an individual situation.

Consolidated Omnibus Reconciliation Act

By the mid-1980s, Congress began to address some of the problems associated with the American employer-based health insurance system. If a worker with employer paid health insurance benefits stopped working for any reason, access to health care was jeopardized for the worker and his or her dependents, putting the health of many individuals at risk. Enacted in 1986, COBRA goes a long way toward eliminating these problems for most, but not all, employees who receive health benefits from their employers (3).

COBRA does this by providing certain former employees, retirees, spouses, former spouses, and dependent children, known as *qualified beneficiaries*, the right to a temporary continuation of their group health insurance coverage at group rates even if their employment or life situation changes. This *COBRA continuation of coverage* is only available when coverage is lost due to certain specific events, known as *qualifying events*, such as a job change, divorce, or becoming eligible for Medicare. COBRA coverage is more expensive than the health insurance coverage paid for by active employees because the employer typically pays the lion's share of the premium for their active employees and dependents and the entire premium must be paid by the former employee under COBRA. The former employee pays 100 percent of his or her premium, plus a 2 percent administration fee. Note that due to differences in the claims experience or risks of each group, health plans' premium amounts vary even when they offer comparable benefits or are provided by the same insurer. As expensive as COBRA premiums may seem, however, they are likely much lower in cost than premiums for an individual (nongroup) health insurance policy, and they are extremely important for maintaining access to health care.

Eligibility for COBRA Continuation of Coverage

COBRA generally covers health plans maintained by private sector employers with 20 or more employees, unions, and employers in state or local governments. Federal employees are covered by a law that is comparable to COBRA, and readers should contact their agency's personnel office for details. Additionally, most states have enacted laws to provide workers of even smaller employers with some rights to continued health benefits. Note that these so-called "mini-COBRA" laws vary significantly from state to state, and details can be obtained from the employer or from state departments of insurance or insurance commissions.

To be eligible for COBRA, an individual must have been enrolled in an employer's group health plan when the qualifying event occurred, and the plan must continue to be in effect for active employees. In the event of a bankruptcy, health plans are terminated and the law does not provide former employees with any contingency for continued or replacement health coverage. COBRA benefits do not begin automatically, and qualified individuals must formally "elect" their COBRA rights. The law requires employers or health plan administrators to notify employees of their COBRA rights on two occasions—when they first enroll in the health plan and again within a specified number of days from the qualifying event. Specific details such as the number of days one has to elect COBRA, the length of COBRA coverage, the number of days former employers have to notify qualified beneficiaries of their rights, and so on vary depending on the qualifying event and other factors. This information should be well-understood by anyone who hopes to take advantage of COBRA's provisions. The key source of information specific to any qualified individual's rights is the health plan itself, although, as the regulatory agency that oversees COBRA, the United States Department of Labor also provides comprehensive information (www.dol.gov/edsa/faqs/faq_consumer_cobra.html).

Qualifying Events

Qualifying events for employees are (a) termination of employment (either voluntary or involuntary as long as there is no gross misconduct involved) and (b) a reduction in the number of working hours making an employee no longer eligible for the employer health plan. Qualifying events for spouses are:

- Voluntary or involuntary termination of a covered employee's employment
- Reduction in the work hours of the covered employee
- Covered employee becoming entitled to Medicare
- Divorce or legal separation from the covered employee
- Death of the covered employee

Qualifying events for dependent children are the same as for spouses, but they include an additional, very significant one for young adults, namely, the loss of dependent child status under the health plan's rules.

Example 1

Nathan, who has been living with MS for 22 years, plans to retire on or about his sixty-fifth birthday when he will become eligible for Medicare. But Nathan's wife, Audrey, also gets her health insurance from Nathan's employer and won't turn 65 until 2 years later. Nathan talks it over with someone in his personnel department, who assures him that Audrey will be eligible for a continuation of their current health coverage for approximately $425 per month. Nathan and Audrey adapt their retirement plans to factor in the additional $10,000 it will cost them to maintain Audrey's coverage over a 2-year period.

COBRA's Start and Stop Dates

COBRA imposes responsibilities on both employers and qualified beneficiaries. For example, beneficiaries must notify their employers (or the employer's plan administrator if they use one) when a qualifying event has occurred, and the employers must inform the beneficiaries of their right to COBRA's continuation of benefits including deadlines for electing COBRA, the amount of the premium, and payment schedule. Each qualified beneficiary may independently elect COBRA coverage, and initial payments are due within 45 days of the election. COBRA coverage technically begins the first day that group coverage would otherwise have ended, so there should be no disruption in coverage for any qualified beneficiary.

118

The amount of time anyone can maintain COBRA continuation, known as the *qualifying period*, depends on the qualifying event that led to his or her electing COBRA initially. When the event is termination of employment, or becoming ineligible for the plan due to a reduction in work hours, the qualifying period is 18 months. All other qualifying events, that is, divorce, legal separation, death of the employee, becoming eligible for Medicare, and "aging out" of a parent's health plan, the qualifying period is 36 months.

An important later addition to the law helps workers who become disabled and apply for Social Security Disability Insurance (SSDI) after leaving work. If the date the Social Security Administration (SSA) determines the disability existed is within the first 60 days of COBRA, then all of the qualified individuals may extend their COBRA coverage for an additional 11 months. It is critical that the employee provides the SSA notice of disability to their employer in order to obtain this extension. In effect, the law treats the onset of disability as a separate qualifying event. However, the employer or plan administrator may increase the premium for the additional 11 months of coverage by an (often unaffordable) 50 percent. This change in COBRA law also recognized other multiple qualifying events, such as a divorce taking place while one is already on COBRA, thus triggering a second qualifying period. In no case, however, may qualifying periods exceed 36 months.

Example 2

Judy's MS-related fatigue worsened dramatically with her last exacerbation. She decides not to return to work, and her employer formally terminates her employment on March 30, 2007. She uses that date on her application for Social Security Disability Insurance benefits where it asks her when the disability began. Because her husband's health plan does not cover dependents, she elects her COBRA benefits, which cost her $374 per month. Approximately 6 months after she filed the application, Judy receives notice from the SSA that she has been approved for benefits, and that her disability began on March 30, 2007. However, she will not become eligible for Medicare until September 2009, a full 29 months after her disability began. With no better option for securing health coverage until then, Judy sends a copy of the SSA's notice to her former employer and tells them she will probably stay on COBRA coverage until her Medicare coverage begins in 2009. Fearful that after 18 months her employer will increase her COBRA premium to $561 as the employer is legally entitled to do, Judy includes a letter describing their circumstances and requesting an exception be made. Her former employer calls her to let her know that they have agreed not to increase her premium above the $374 she pays during the first 18 months.

Beware of Waiting Periods

Most people use their COBRA privileges to maintain coverage for some period of time as they move from one health plan to another, such as when changing jobs. When planning to make a transition from one employer's group health plan to another, it is important to know that some group health plans require a *waiting period* for all new group plan members. Simply put, waiting periods are a specified amount of time (typically 1 to 3 months) that newly eligible individuals must wait before their enrollment into a new health plan becomes effective. Health maintenance organizations may use the term *affiliation period* instead. As the next example shows, to assure a smooth transition in coverage with no breaks in coverage, it is best to maintain one's COBRA benefits through the waiting period (if there is one). The *effective date* of coverage typically occurs the first day of the month following the end of a newly eligible individual's waiting period.

Example 3

Cassandra gives her current employer notice that she will be leaving her job on June 15. She has already accepted a new position to begin on July 9. Even though her new employer also offers health coverage, there is a 3- month waiting period for all new employees, so she would not be covered by the new plan until November 1. To assure that she does not go without health coverage for even 1 day, she elects her COBRA benefits and pays her former employer $513 per month in August, September,and October.

Benefits and Claims Filing Under COBRA

The good news for all three of the individuals described in the examples above is that the benefits of their COBRA plan must be identical to those offered to active employees and others in the employee health plan. Unfortunately, that also means that if the benefits are changed in some way for all plan members, such as increases in the prescription drug copayment amounts, those increases must be borne by people on COBRA as well. Claims are filed in the exact same way as an active employee, and the same procedures are in force regarding appeals for any claims that are denied by the health plan. Finally, a note of caution about COBRA benefits. It is important for people on COBRA to pay their premiums on time and to assume that a late payment can jeopardize their continued enrollment in the plan. Employers and plan administrators are not required by law to send bills or payment reminders, so anyone on COBRA needs to be mindful of their payment obligations and due dates.

Health Insurance Portability and Accountability Act

The Clinton Administration's attempt to reform the health care system and provide health coverage for all Americans never garnered enough support from congressional lawmakers to become law. But the debate surrounding that initiative heightened awareness of the unresolved problems in America's employer-based health care system (4). It was this awareness that created the political will necessary to enact a complex federal law to expand protections against discrimination in health insurance, particularly for people with preexisting health conditions. That legislation was called the Health Insurance Portability and Accountability Act of 1996, also known as HIPAA.

Although COBRA effectively eliminated the likelihood of becoming uninsured as a result of common life or workplace changes, prior to HIPAA there was no guarantee that new employees and their dependents would automatically be accepted into an employer's health plan, especially if one or more family members had a preexisting health condition. The demand for *portability* of health coverage, or the ability to maintain one's eligibility for coverage, became the focal point of HIPAA legislation.

Prior to HIPAA, all health insurance plans could effectively screen out potential new plan members with high health care costs by refusing to cover any with preexisting health conditions, or by limiting the policies in other ways to avoid responsibility for major medical bills. With no legal restrictions on these practices, insurers were free to write their own rules in ways designed to minimize their losses at the expense of people the insurance industry deemed high risks. Even women of child-bearing age, those in high-risk occupations, those who enjoyed contact sports, long-term survivors of childhood diseases, or the "near elderly" were singled out and denied health plan enrollment or penalized through higher premiums. HIPAA ended these practices by standardizing the rules under which all group health plans must operate, and leveling the playing field for most, but not all, health plans.

121

Much to the frustration of advocates for the chronically ill and disabled, HIPAA's strongest protections serve workers and their dependents covered through *group* health plans and provide only marginal help for the self-employed and anyone ineligible for group health benefits. Like COBRA, the rights and responsibilities HIPAA imposes on plans and plan members are complex, and I will use some specific case examples to better understand those rights and responsibilities. Also, like COBRA, the focus of HIPAA is to gain or maintain eligibility for health insurance, but unfortunately it does little to make health insurance more affordable (3).

HIPAA's Nondiscrimination Provisions

HIPAA prohibits all group health plans of two or more members from denying enrollment to anyone on the basis of their health status or history of preexisting health problems. It also assures that no plan member can be singled out and charged a higher premium or be treated differently than any other member. So, if the plan requires a 25 percent coinsurance for injectible drugs, it must do so for all members. HIPAA also guarantees that all group health plans must be renewable, including small groups with high medical expenses.

Preexisting Condition Defined

As previously noted, excluding the costs associated with a person's preexisting condition had been one of the insurance industry's methods for avoiding high medical costs. In a compromise with health plans, HIPAA allows the industry to continue excluding preexisting conditions, but strictly limits the length of the exclusion period to 1 year or 18 months, depending on how quickly an individual becomes enrolled.

HIPAA also standardizes the definition of a *preexisting condition* as "any condition, whether physical or mental, regardless of the cause of the condition, for which medical advice, diagnosis, care or treatment is recommended or received within the six-month period ending on the enrollment date." Put more simply, a preexisting condition is one for which a person has received care within 6 months prior to joining the health plan. It is important to understand that taking medication qualifies as treatment even if the patient did not see a doctor during that time period. Once enrolled in the plan, however, any new condition or treatment is covered even if it began during a waiting period if the health plan has one.

122

Limits on Preexisting Condition Exclusions

The maximum amount of time a group health plan can exclude coverage for a preexisting condition is 365 days (12 months) when a new plan member enrolls during his or her *initial enrollment period*, or 546 days (18 months) for anyone who delays enrollment until later. This disparity points out one of HIPAA's built-in incentives for eligible individuals to participate in the health insurance system.

The value of HIPAA's rule limiting preexisting condition exclusions becomes clearer if we compare someone with a relatively inexpensive preexisting condition to a person who has highly expensive treatment costs. Let's say a new plan enrollee with insomnia learns her new plan considers the insomnia a preexisting condition and will not cover the costs of her prescription medication for the first year she is in the plan. Paying $127 for the monthly refills of her sleeping medication will probably be affordable for her for that year, and could probably be absorbed, even if she had to continue paying beyond that time. HIPAA is helpful to her, but would probably not be a determinant of whether she continues her medication or not. For a person with MS, however, where treatment costs can reach tens of thousands of dollars per year, the ability of an enrollee to cover this cost beyond a 1-year exclusion period would probably be impossible. Therefore, HIPAA protections are extremely important when insured individuals have expensive health conditions.

Creditable Coverage Provides Portability of Coverage

Another goal of HIPAA is to make sure that individuals with preexisting conditions only have to meet that exclusion period once. It does this through the concept of *creditable coverage*. If you have met the exclusion period with one group health plan, and receive a certificate of creditable coverage to prove it, this provides credit toward the exclusion period of any new health plan you join. So, anyone who has at least 12 months of creditable coverage from a previous plan cannot have any costs associated with a preexisting condition excluded from their coverage in a new plan. Creditable coverage can also be reached by combining the months from an old and new plan. This means if you bring 6 months of creditable coverage to a health plan, you only need 6 months in that new plan before your exclusion period is over.

However, not all prior health coverage is considered creditable coverage and subject to HIPAA's portability provisions. Coverage from any group or individual health plan, Medicare, Medicaid, plans provided by the military, Indian Health Service or Peace Corps, the federal employees' plan, state high-risk pools, and public health plans all qualify as creditable coverage and are therefore portable when enrolling in a new group health plan. Disability, long-term care and life insurance, worker's compensation, disease-specific or catastrophic health insurance, Medicare supplemental plans, some student policies, and temporary health insurance do not qualify and have no portability to a future health plan.

Example 1

Amanda was adequately covered by her husband Bill's employer health plan for 7 years before they moved to California when Bill was offered a job with another architectural firm. The new firm offered health benefits to both employees and their dependents, but they worried about the exclusion for preexisting conditions since Amanda was diagnosed with MS 2 years ago. But Bill's personnel office assured him that the time Amanda was covered under Bill's old plan could be applied to the 12 month preexisting condition exclusion period of the new plan.

Example 2

Helen's first job out of college was in a department store, and she was glad they provided health benefits. But a better job opportunity came along and she gave her notice after only 6 months on the job. She started the new job right away and signed up for her new employer's health plan. But the first time she submitted a claim for her prescription refills, the claim was denied. Her Human Resources Director explained that any costs associated with a preexisting condition would be excluded from her coverage for up to a year, but that any amount of time she had been covered by her previous employer's plan would count toward that 12- month exclusion. So, after 6 months in her new plan, Helen's medications for her MS were covered. Before the 6 months were up, Helen had an accident on her bicycle and went to the emergency room for x-rays. Because none of the costs she incurred in the emergency room were related to a preexisting condition, her plan covered them all.

Demonstrating Creditable Coverage

As the examples above suggest, all group health plans have the right to determine whether a new plan member has a preexisting condition and to review details of their creditable coverage. To facilitate this information sharing and protect portability rights, HIPAA requires all group health plans to provide an individualized *Certificate of Creditable Coverage* to former group plan members. This certificate must be provided either upon the request of the qualified beneficiary, when the COBRA election notice is provided, or within a reasonable time after COBRA coverage ceases. Many people receive their certificate of creditable coverage in the mail, or along with other documents they receive as they leave their jobs, not realizing how important it may be in assuring a seamless transition into full coverage with their new group. It is strongly recommended that people with expensive preexisting health conditions in particular pay attention to their Certificate of Creditable Coverage and keep it in a safe and accessible location. If the certificate is not available, proof of prior coverage may be provided with the membership card of the former health plan or copies of paid medical bills.

HIPAA's Portability Protections are Lost Unless Coverage is Maintained

It is important to understand HIPAA as powerful legal protection against the potentially harsh consequences of a health plan's preexisting condition exclusion, but one that comes with a price. Prior coverage is not creditable if there is a break in coverage for 63 or more days, thus establishing another of HIPAA's built-in incentives to stay insured. Even if a person was securely insured for years, but experienced a sudden change in circumstances leading to their loss of health insurance for 63 days or more, none of his or her prior coverage is considered creditable and, therefore, portable to any future health plan's preexisting exclusion period. Because of this fact, it is crucial that people who have ongoing health conditions do not have a lapse in coverage. This makes the COBRA benefit particularly important. As expensive as COBRA premiums may seem, it is likely less expensive for people with MS to elect COBRA than it is to suffer the consequences of a preexisting condition exclusion in the future. The following examples help make these points.

Example 3

Wendie had always been covered by her husband Stephen's employer plan, but they went through some very hard times after he was laid off. Although eligible for COBRA, the premium for both of them to stay on the plan would have been over $800 per month. Their priority was keeping Wendie on the plan to maintain her access to her MS medications and care by her neurologist. So Wendie elected her COBRA continuation benefits at a cost of $413 per month, and Stephen declined it. Fortunately, Stephen found new employment within about 5 months, and he quickly enrolled them both in the new employer's plan. Wendie suffered no exclusion for her preexisting MS, and Stephen had no preexisting condition to be excluded anyway. Both were adequately covered with no disruption to Wendie's care.

Example 4

Arthur felt extremely grateful to have the health benefits his engineering firm provided to him and his dependents, especially after his daughter Chloe was diagnosed with MS at age 17. But tragedy struck when the firm was found liable in a major lawsuit and had to file for bankruptcy. Although Arthur, his family, and most of his former colleagues suddenly found themselves with no health coverage, Arthur was confident that the situation was temporary, as he was interviewing for new jobs within a matter of months. Arthur did secure new employment within that time span, but the 137 day gap in health insurance meant that none of the costs of Chloe's MS-related care would be covered for the first 12 months she was covered under her father's new policy.

HIPAA's Assistance for Individuals

As previously noted, HIPAA's portability provisions are only applicable to new group health plan enrollees. That leaves *individual* insurance, which is commercially sold nongroup health insurance, outside the scope of HIPAA and, as a result, more a matter of state law than federal. But Congress did address the needs of individuals with preexisting health conditions by requiring the states to assure that any of their residents who meet certain criteria must be able to buy an individual health insurance policy of some kind without a preexisting condition exclusion. HIPAA standardized the criteria for the right to an individual policy, and individuals are *HIPAA eligible* only if they meet the following criteria:

1. Eighteen months of continuous creditable coverage, the last day of which was under a group health plan
2. COBRA or other continuation benefit has been exhausted
3. Ineligibility for group health insurance, Medicaid, or Medicare
4. No current health insurance coverage
5. Application within 63 days of the termination of prior coverage

126

States have complied with, and at times expanded upon, this requirement in various ways, including high-risk pools, guaranteed issue plans, and COBRA conversion policies. An excellent state-by-state source on what is available in each state is available on-line at www.healthinsuranceinfo.net.

HIPAA Protects Private Medical Information

The last major set of HIPAA provisions to be fully implemented through regulation addresses rights and responsibilities regarding *protected health information*. This includes all information in patient records, conversations between providers and payers (insurance or government programs) regarding a patient's health care, and billing information. Providers and insurers must assure that patients have the ability to see and get copies of their records, make corrections to their records, receive notice describing how protected health information may be used, and understand their right to control how and when their information is shared with others. The use and exchange of protected health information can be particularly important for people with MS and other chronic health conditions to facilitate and coordinate their care, for use in research, and to ensure its accuracy and the proper administration of benefits and payments. The privacy portion of HIPAA is regulated by the Office of Civil Rights in the United States Health and Human Services Administration, and additional information may be obtained online at www.hhs.gov/ocr/hipaa or by calling 1-866-627-7748.

Family and Medical Leave Act

So far, this chapter has been a discussion of federal laws focused primarily on health insurance benefits provided by employers—always an important issue for working-age people with chronic health conditions. Signed into law in 1993, the FMLA also protects health benefits, but is thought of primarily as a law protecting one's employment during a health care crisis experienced by a worker or family member (5,6). Under FMLA, eligible workers are allowed to take up to a total of 12 work weeks of unpaid leave during a 12-month period, with continued health benefits, for one or more of the following reasons (6):

- The birth and care of the employee's newborn child
- Placement with the employee of a child for adoption or foster care

127

- To care for an immediate family member (spouse, child, or parent) with a serious health condition
- To take medical leave when the employee is unable to work because of a serious health condition

FMLA applies to nearly all employers, including state, local and federal government agencies, schools, and private-sector employers who have had 50 or more employees on the payroll for 20 work weeks during the current or preceding calendar year. Any employee who meets the following criteria is eligible for family and medical leave:

1. Employed by the employer for at least 12 months (not necessarily consecutively)
2. Worked a minimum of 1,250 hours during the last year
3. Works at a worksite that has 50 or more employees (or employs 50 or more people within 75 miles using surface transportation)

The FMLA does not provide paid leave, and employers can require (or permit) an employee to use all available accrued but unused vacation, sick, or paid time off (PTO) time during such leave. If employees use paid vacation, personal, or other leave during their 12-week leave, it will count against the 12-week maximum amount of time they are entitled to be on leave under the FMLA. If workers qualify for disability insurance benefits, they are entitled to receive it while on FMLA. Still, surveys show that many people who experience medical or caretaking emergencies do not take a leave because they cannot afford to forfeit their income at the same time.

Preparing to Take Medical Leave

Generally, it is the employee's responsibility to give notice of the need for a medical leave, which may be given in person or by phone or other electronic means. Someone acting on the employee's behalf may also give the notice. Employees who experience the need for a leave should not assume that they have satisfied their responsibility to give their employer notice of their need to take leave by simply not returning to work. The notice must be provided at least 30 days in advance when the need is foreseeable or as soon as practicable when the need for leave is not foreseeable.

Families affected by MS who take advantage of the FMLA may be less able to plan their leave, since most will likely need it following an acute exacerbation. Nonetheless, it is wise for workers or family members to work with the employer to avoid disruptions to the workplace as much as possible. Employees do not have to provide medical records to an employer to justify an FMLA leave, although employers may require something from a doctor to certify that a serious health condition exists. This could include a description of the health condition plus dates and expected duration of the treatment plan.

Example 1

Sandy suffers a major exacerbation of her MS symptoms and is admitted to the hospital. Her daughter, Beth, lives in a town nearby and acts as her advocate with Sandy's doctors, insurers, and others. Although Sandy will be released back to her own home in 48 hours, her doctor prescribes a course of physical and occupational therapy for the next month. Beth calls Sandy's employer to give them notice that her mother will require a medical leave for 5 weeks starting immediately. Then Beth calls her own employer to notify them that she will be taking 2 weeks of medical leave to stay with her mother during her most fragile phase. Her personnel manager reminds her that under their policy, employees must use up any vacation or sick days before they can take unpaid family or medical leave, and Beth still has 4 vacation days left that year. Beth still takes 2 weeks away from work, including 4 vacation days and 6 days under FMLA.

Guaranteed Ability to Return to the Same Job and Maintenance of Health Benefits

With an exception for some key employees (i.e., the highest paid 10 percent of workers), the FMLA requires that the employee must be returned to the same or equivalent position on return from leave. The equivalent position provision is strict, and includes pay, benefits, privileges, and any other terms or conditions of employment (7). For example, if the employer offers a perfect attendance bonus, the FMLA cannot be used as a basis for denying the bonus. However, if an eligible employee needs to take medical leave on an intermittent basis, say for days or even hours at a time, the employer may require him or her to temporarily transfer to another position at the same pay and benefits if it is better suited for recurring periods of leave. The law also requires employers to maintain

129

any health benefits during the leave that are normally provided to the employee while they are working.

Example 1

Michelle's MS has been worsening in the past year. Between the fall she took in March and a case of the flu in June, she had used up all of her paid leave (sick and vacation days). She suffered a major exacerbation in July and took 9 weeks of unpaid medical leave, then took the remaining 3 weeks of medical leave she was entitled to in October. When she didn't feel capable of returning to work at the beginning of November, however, she asked her employer for an extension on her FMLA. Although sympathetic, her employer could not have Michelle absent from her position any longer, and Michelle lost her job. With help from her parents, she was able to afford her COBRA premiums to maintain her health coverage, and began the process of applying for disability insurance benefits from the Social Security Administration.

State FMLA Laws

It is important for readers to know that as of 2007, 11 states had enacted laws similar to, but often more generous than, the federal FMLA. For example, eligible California residents can get paid during a medical leave under certain circumstances. The U.S. Department of Labor maintains detailed information comparing all of the state laws to the federal FMLA. These comparisons can be viewed online at www.dol.gov/esa/programs/whd/state/fmla/index, or by calling the Wage and Hour Division of the U.S. Department of Labor at 1-866-487-9243. Covered employers must comply with whatever federal or state provision provides the greater benefit to their employees, although the U.S. Department of Labor can only enforce the federal law, and states must enforce their own laws.

Summary

Three important federal laws were passed between the years 1986 and 1996 giving new rights to workers, and they are of particular importance to people living with a chronic health condition. Designed to help people maintain their employer-based health insurance coverage, COBRA and HIPAA can be critical to individuals or families living with MS. The key to making best use of their many protections is to understand how they relate to one's particular circumstances. Good basic planning and access to accurate information about COBRA and HIPAA allow workers and their families to transition through job changes, a divorce, early retirement, or other changing circumstances without fear of losing their access to health care. Likewise, the FMLA provides eligible workers with the security of knowing their jobs and benefits will be waiting for them if or when a medical leave is necessary.

References

1. Enthoven, A.C., & Fuchs, V.R. (2006). Employment-based health insurance: Past, present, and future. *Health Affairs, 25*(6), 1538–1547.
2. Moran, D.W. (2005). Whence and whither health insurance? A revisionist history. *Health Affairs, 24*(6), 1415–1425.
3. Garner, J.C. (2001). *Health insurance answer book.* 6th Edition. New York: Panel Publishers.
4. Iglehart, J.K. (2005). The struggle that never ends: Reforming U.S. health care. *Health Affairs, 24*(6), 1396–1397.
5. Northrop, S.C., Cooper, S.E., & Calder, K.C. (2007). *Health insurance resources: A guide for people with chronic disease and disability.* 2nd Edition. New York: Demos Medical Publishing.
6. Rumrill, P., & Hennessey, M. (2001) *Multiple sclerosis: A guide for healthcare and rehabilitation professionals.* Springfield, IL: Charles C Thomas.

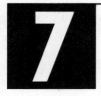

Social Security Disability Benefits

Steven W. Nissen

Phillip D. Rumrill, Jr.

Mary L. Hennessey

E VEN WITH THE MYRIAD of services, resources, and legal protections that are available to help people with multiple sclerosis (MS) obtain and maintain employment, there may come a time when the individual with MS decides that it is time to leave the work force. It is important to explore all employment options and protections before prematurely taking this step. Such persons will hopefully have utilized reasonable accommodations under the Americans with Disabilities Act (ADA), the Family and Medical Leave Act (FMLA), and any other legal protections designed to help themselves stay in the workplace as long as possible. Once they decide to leave the work force, they may consider applying for disability benefits from the Social Security Administration (SSA). This chapter will address the different types of disability benefits available from SSA, the process a person has to go through in order to apply for benefits, and what options a person has to work once he or she has been awarded benefits. The chapter will also explain the different types of health insurance available through Social Security; namely, Medicare and Medicaid. Work incentives and apparent disincentives will also be discussed—inherent risks or concerns that individuals with MS experience once on Social Security when and if they attempt to return to work. These include loss of financial benefits and health insurance coverage.

133

Disability Determinations

SSA has a strict definition of disability that must be met in order to be awarded disability benefits. The definition of disability:

> is based on your inability to work. We consider you disabled under Social Security rules if you cannot do work that you did before and we decide that you cannot adjust to other work because of your medical condition(s). Your disability must also last or be expected to last for at least 1 year or to result in death (1, p.11).

For people with MS, meeting that definition of disability under the SSA system can be difficult due to the variability and unpredictability of the symptoms, as well as the often invisible symptoms a person with MS may experience. The SSA publishes a manual entitled *Disability Evaluation Under Social Security* (2), also known as the "Blue Book," which is written primarily for health care providers and professionals to clarify the Social Security process and the symptoms SSA is looking for in determining disability for various types of medical conditions. In the Blue Book (3), MS is listed under adult neurological conditions (section 11.00) and is further described in section 11.09(4). This section describes the symptoms of multiple sclerosis that the SSA recognizes as (2):

1. Disorganization of motor function as described in 11.04B
2. Visual or mental impairment as described under the criteria in 2.02, 2.03, 2.04, or 12.02
3. Significant, reproducible fatigue of motor function with substantial muscle weakness on repetitive activity, demonstrated on physical examination, resulting from neurological dysfunction in areas of the central nervous system known to be pathologically involved by the multiple sclerosis process

An individual with MS must demonstrate symptoms with motor function or gait difficulties, visual or mental symptoms (including cognition), and/or fatigue with muscle weakness. Of course, these areas of functional limitation reflect the most commonly observed effects of MS (see Chapter 1). Even so, because several of these symptoms are hard to objectively describe or assess, the process a person with MS goes through in documenting his or her disability may be challenging and difficult.

When a person with MS does decide to apply for Social Security, it is important that the doctors, especially the treating neurologist, are aware of this decision. Medical records and documentation will be obtained by SSA in order for them to review the application. If the doctor clearly states the impact that the MS symptoms are having on the individual's ability to work at a competitive and productive level, it will help the individual through the application process. The more descriptive and detailed the records are, the fewer questions SSA's disability determination unit may have to ask to evaluate the claim.

Supplemental Security Income and Social Security Disability Insurance

There are two different disability programs—Supplemental Security Income (SSI) and Social Security Disability Insurance (SSDI). For both programs, the individual must meet the definition of disability as previously described. The main difference between the two programs is that SSI is based on (a) financial need and (b) intended for the individual who has not worked the necessary number of credits (or quarters) and, therefore, has not contributed the required money to the Social Security system. SSI is supported by general tax revenues and not by earmarked Social Security taxes. According to SSA, it is primarily intended to help aged, blind, and disabled people who have little or no income, and in essence, SSI is for people who are too disabled to work, poor, and who have limited recent work histories (5).

SSDI is based on an individual's prior work history and is the federal disability insurance policy. SSDI is awarded for total disability—no benefits are awarded for partial disability or for conditions that are expected to last only a short time. The individual must meet the definition of disability described earlier. This disability benefit is for people who have a significant work history. To be eligible for SSDI, in addition to meeting the definition of disability, one must have worked long enough—and recently enough—under Social Security to qualify for disability benefits. Social Security work credits are based on one's total yearly wages or self-employment income. A person can earn up to four credits each year, one for each 3-month quarter of the calendar year. The amount of earnings needed for a credit changes from year to year. In 2007, for example, the person earns one credit for each $1000 of wages or self-employment income. When a person has earned $4,000, he or she has earned the requisite four credits for the year. The number of work credits one needs to qualify for

SSDI benefits depends on age, and when the person becomes disabled. Generally, SSDI applicants need 40 credits, 20 of which were earned in the last 10 years before he or she became disabled (6). To apply for SSDI, the individual must not be working at all or working below a figure known as the Substantial Gainful Activity (SGA) level. The SGA is the figure that SSA determines to represent being "competitively employed."

If the person has a recent-enough and long-enough work history, then they have been contributing to the Social Security system. When people are working for wages, the amount due the SSA system has been taken out of their pay as FICA contributions. This amount of money has been put into the Social Security "trust fund" for the future. When a person is receiving SSDI, money is being withdrawn that has been deposited into this monetary pool under his or her name.

The vast majority of Americans with MS have employment histories, and most were working at the time of diagnosis. Therefore, many individuals with MS may be eligible for SSDI based on having worked a significant number of years. This is not always the case, but people with MS receive SSDI benefits more often than they receive SSI. It is important to keep in mind that SSDI applications require a 5-month waiting period from the determination of disability to the start of benefits. SSI does not have any waiting period and benefits begin upon determination of disability and financial need.

The Process

An application for Social Security can be made in several ways. Applicants can contact the SSA at 1-800-772-1213 and complete an application over the telephone. They can also go in person to a local Social Security Administration field office. Readers may locate their local office online by going to https://secure.ssa.gov/apps6z/FOLO/fo001.jsp and entering their zip code. Applicants can also apply for disability benefits on-line at www.socialsecurity.gov/applyfordisability/. All applicants must complete the application as well as the Adult Disability Report.

For most individuals who are applying for SSDI, the process can be time consuming and frustrating. Most applications for disability, regardless of the medical condition, are denied at the initial application. This is often the case for individuals with MS. Once a person applies for disability benefits and an initial decision has been made, he or she will receive notification in writing from the SSA. As mentioned previously, more often than not, the individual with MS will be denied benefits at the initial application. The individual will be given 60 days to appeal that decision, and it is generally suggested that the individual appeal because appeals are granted at a higher rate than original applications. During that first appeal, the claim is assigned to a representative from the SSA who was not involved in the original decision. The individual will again receive written notification as to whether the claim has been denied or approved. If denied, the applicant will be given another 60 days to appeal that decision. The third appeal will be brought before an administrative law judge. Up until this point, decisions on the claim have been made by the disability determination office based on the paper file. At this third appeal, the claimant goes before a judge who has the authority to award or deny benefits. According to Northrop et al. (7), this is similar to a court hearing or trial, but less formal. Testimony is taken under oath, and the parties are permitted to submit evidence. If the claimant is denied at this stage, he or she can request a review by the Social Security Appeals Council in Washington, DC, within 60 days of the date of the determination by the judge. If the client disagrees with the Appeal Council's decision, or the Appeal Council refuses to hear the claim, there is one more appeal that can be made. The claimant can file a civil suit in federal district court (8). It should be noted that all Social Security applicants have the right to legal representation from the very beginning of the disability determination process. In fact, we strongly recommend that readers retain Social Security attorneys for all appeals and reconsiderations because having legal representation increases one's chances of prevailing at all levels of review.

When considering an application for disability benefits from Social Security, it is important to keep in mind the time it may take to be approved for benefits. It can take anywhere from a few months to over a year to be awarded benefits from the SSA. The applicant should plan for a possible period of unemployment. Planning ahead is critical. By virtue of applying for SSDI, the person must prove that he or she is not able to work. It is important to consider how bills are going to continue to be paid. Therefore, financial planning must be part of the master plan.

Health Insurance Options: Medicaid and Medicare

Health insurance coverage is often a major concern for persons with MS. For those receiving benefits from Social Security, health insurance coverage is included, but it differs based on the type of benefit the person

137

is receiving. For the SSI recipient, Medicaid is the insurance coverage available. For the SSDI recipient, Medicare is the insurance coverage.

Medicaid coverage begins immediately when SSI benefits begin. According to *The Medicaid Resource Book* (9, p. 50), "Most Medicaid beneficiaries are entitled to coverage for the following basic services, if the services are medically necessary:

- Hospital care (inpatient and outpatient)
- Nursing home care
- Physician services
- Laboratory and x-ray services
- Immunizations and other early and periodic screening, diagnostic, and treatment services for children
- Family planning services
- Health center and rural health clinic services
- Nurse midwife and nurse practitioner services"

States have the *option* of offering certain additional services through Medicaid. States can receive federal matching funds for these added services (9, p. 50):

- Prescription drugs
- Institutional care for individuals with mental retardation
- Home- and community-based care for the frail elderly, including case management
- Personal care and other community-based services for individuals with disabilities
- Dental care and vision care for adults

The Centers for Medicare and Medicaid Services administer Medicare, the nation's largest health insurance program, which covers nearly 40 million Americans. Medicare is available for people 65 years of age and older, some people with disabilities under 65 years of age, and people with end-stage renal disease (i.e., permanent kidney failure treated with dialysis or a transplant) (10). Although Medicare is administered by the Centers for Medicare and Medicaid Services, the application for receiving Medicare must be filed with the SSA.

Individuals who have been deemed disabled by the SSA and have been receiving SSDI benefits for 24 months are eligible for Medicare.

This means that there is a 2-year waiting period before the SSDI recipient will have insurance coverage through Medicare. This is another time where the person should plan ahead as to how to maintain health insurance coverage during this period. As described in Chapter 6, individuals may be able to extend their COBRA coverage for up to 36 months if they are Medicare eligible. This is an important option to consider if people can afford the premiums that would allow their health insurance benefits to continue until Medicare takes effect.

Medicare has four parts (11):

- Hospital insurance (Part A) that helps pay for inpatient care in a hospital or skilled nursing facility (following a hospital stay), some home health care, and hospice care.
- Medical insurance (Part B) that helps pay for physicians' services and many other medical services and supplies that are not covered by hospital insurance.
- Medicare Advantage (Part C), formerly known as Medicare + Choice, plans are available in many areas. People with Medicare Parts A and B can choose to receive all of their health care services through a provider organization, such as health maintenance organizations (HMOs), perferred provider organizations (PPOs), or other service providers.
- Prescription drug coverage (Part D) that helps pay for medications that physicians prescribe for treatment.

Part A comes automatically and free of charge for most Medicare recipients. Part B and Part D are optional. One must elect to have this coverage and there are premiums affiliated with the coverage. The premiums for these plans vary each year. In 2007, for example, Part B premiums was normally $93.50 per month (this could be more if a person's yearly income is exceptionally high). Part D premiums vary greatly by state and by type of coverage provided (e.g., how large the deductible is, coverage gaps). In 2007, the national average premium for Part D was $27.35 per month.

For both Part B and Part D, one will face a financial penalty for not enrolling when first eligible for coverage, then later deciding to enroll, unless there is proof of having other creditable coverage that is comparable to or better than what is available from Medicare. The Part B premium may go up 10 percent for each 12-month period that one could have had Medicare Part B but did not take it. This penalty is permanent and must be paid as long as one is covered by Medicare, so it behooves applicants to enroll in Part B as soon as they are eligible for Medicare. With Part D, if one elected not to join when first eligible, upon joining the premium cost will increase at least 1 percent per month for every month that one waited to join. Part D beneficiaries are then required to pay this penalty as long as prescription drug coverage is in effect. Here again, it behooves the applicant to enroll in Part D as soon as he or she becomes eligible for Medicare.

Prescription drug coverage is extremely important to individuals with MS. Part D was first made available in January 2006; prior to that time, those who were on Medicare, either because they were over the age of 65 or receiving SSDI, had no standard prescription drug benefit available to them through the Medicare program. Under Part D, private drug companies that have been approved by Medicare administer the plans. Plans cover different drugs, brand name and/or generic, and maintain their own formulary of covered drugs. They also differ in the cost of premiums, in required deductibles, and in coverage offered.

The following is an outline of the annual costs to the beneficiary of the standard Medicare Part D coverage (7):

● A monthly premium.
● An annual deductible of $265.
● Once the deductible is paid, the beneficiary pays 25 percent copay for all drugs covered in the selected Part D plan until the total prescription drug costs reaches $2,400.
● All prescription drug costs from this point on are the responsibility of the beneficiary until the total drug costs reach $5,451.
● The beneficiary pays 5 percent of covered drug costs after the cumulative costs have reached $5,451.

This process repeats annually.

Importantly, the gap in coverage for medications with annual costs of $2,400 to $5,451 is known as the "donut hole" (7). This gap is a basic component of virtually every Part D plan. Beneficiaries must continue to pay their monthly premium even while the donut hole requires them to pay all of the costs of their medications. The catastrophic coverage component begins once the beneficiary has incurred more than $5,451 in total drug costs in a calendar year (in other words, a maximum of $3,850 in out-of-pocket costs), at which point the beneficiary pays only 5 percent of future drug costs. The Medicare Part D plan is responsible for keeping track of enrollees' cumulative costs (7).

By the time individuals reach catastrophic coverage, they may have paid up to $3,850 out of pocket (deductible, copay amount, and coverage gap). This may be cost prohibitive for some individuals, but given the expense of some MS treatments and medications, it may cost even more to have no coverage at all. These deductibles and copay amounts start over in January of each year.

Some people may be eligible for extra financial help from SSA to cover some of these expenses. Individuals are automatically eligible if they have full coverage under a state Medicaid program as well as Medicare, if they receive assistance from Medicaid for paying Medicare premiums, or they receive SSI. If not automatically eligible, a person can apply for extra help by contacting the SSA at 1-800-772-1213 or by going to www. socialsecurity.gov. If the person is not automatically eligible, SSA will consider assets and income. If the individual's combined savings, investments, and real estate, not including the home, are worth no more than $11,710 if the person is single, or $23,410 if married and living with a spouse, the SSA may grant extra help.

Part D prescription drug plans vary from state to state, as do formularies. It is important to compare plans to determine which one suits the individual's needs. To determine which plan would work best, go to www.medicare. gov and use the Compare Prescription Drug Plans or Formulary Finder options. Input medications, dosage, and preferred pharmacy and obtain a list of prescription drug plans available.

To obtain additional information on Part D, or assistance understanding available plans, contact the State Health Insurance Counseling and Assistance Program at www.healthassistancepartnership.org/ship-locator.

Medicare generally allows for changing one's plan between November 15 and December 31 each year. If eligible for a Medicare Advantage Plan, one may join from January 1 through March 31 each year.

Work Incentives and Disincentives in the Social Security Program

The apparent uncertainty about returning to work evidenced by some persons with MS may be the result of concern that their SSDI or SSI benefits might be withdrawn, thus cutting off stable financial support and health insurance. Given the process that they may have gone through, as described earlier in this chapter, in order to get approved for benefits in the first place, they may not want to do anything that might risk them losing their benefits that they fought long and hard to obtain in the first place.

However, the SSA does offer several work incentives that are designed to assist individuals on SSI or SSDI in their attempt to return to work. Some may be more useful than others to the person with MS who is considering returning to work after being approved for benefits. For the person with MS who is receiving SSDI, there are several work incentives that may be useful to consider—trial work period, substantial gainful activity level, and impairment-related work expenses. SSI beneficiaries derive work incentives from the Plan for Achieving Self Support, and both SSDI and SSI beneficiaries can benefit from the Ticket to Work.

Trial Work Period

According to the SSA's *2007 Red Book* (12), the trial work period (TWP) permits a person receiving SDDI to test his or her ability to work for at least 9 months. During this time, beneficiaries receive *full* SSDI benefits, *regardless of their earnings,* as long as their work activities are reported and they still have disabling impairments. The 9 months do not need to be consecutive and can occur anytime over a 60-month period. Any month where the individual receives more than $640 in wages would count toward the trial work period for 2007. The TWP earnings threshold increases slightly on January 1 of each year due to a cost of living adjustment.

Substantial Gainful Activity

Substantial gainful activity (SGA) level is the figure that SSA considers to represent competitive employment. In order to be eligible for disability benefits, one must demonstrate an inability to work. This means that a person is not working for pay above the SGA level. The SGA is adjusted each January 1, like the trial work period, in accordance with the cost of living. For 2007, the SGA amount for individuals with disabilities other than blindness is $900 per month gross income. For individuals who are deemed blind by SSA, the SGA amount for 2007 is $1500 per month gross income. If an SSDI recipient is working below the SGA amount, and still meets the definition of disability based on his or her medical condition, his or her disability benefits should not be affected.

Impairment-Related Work Expenses

According to the SSA's *2007 Red Book* (12), impairment-related work expenses (IRWE) allow the SSDI recipient to deduct the costs of certain impairment-related items and services that are necessary to maintain employment when determining whether their gross income falls below the allowable SGA level. Importantly, it does not matter if the person uses these impairment-related items and services for his or her personal use outside of work. Let us suppose that a person with MS requires the use of specialized accessible transportation to get to and from work and must pay for this transportation out of his or her pocket. That expense can be deducted from his or her gross income in determining whether he or she complies with the SGA earnings limit. If that person were earning $1000 per month in gross income, and if he or she were paying $200 per month in transportation, his or her actual earnings for purposes of SGA determination would be $800 per month. Other examples of IRWEs can be found in the Social Security *2007 Red Book* (12).

Plan for Achieving Self-Support

The Plan for Achieving Self-Support (PASS) is a work incentive for individuals receiving SSI benefits. With the PASS plan, an SSI recipient creates an individualized plan to achieve specific employment goals. The person sets aside resources and income for a specified period of time to complete education or training, procure work-related equipment, establish a business, or cover any other reasonable expense related to becoming financially self-supporting (13).

Ticket to Work Program

The Ticket to Work program contains a series of incentives for people receiving SSI or SSDI who want to initiate or resume their careers. The Ticket to Work entitles the bearer to a wide range of choices obtaining the employment services, vocational rehabilitation services, and other supports that he or she may need to secure or maintain a job. The Ticket to Work is a free and voluntary program, and beneficiaries who elect not to take advantage of this open-choice service opportunity are not subjected to any penalties or reprisals. Another important feature is that the SSA will not conduct a medical review or reconsideration of one's disability status while he or she is utilizing the Ticket to Work (12). This program is part of the larger Ticket to Work and Work Incentives Improvement Act of 1999 (TWWIIA) which addressed some of the disincentives that were and continue to be inherent to the specter of returning to work and having Social Security's financial and health insurance benefits cease. There are several components of this program that might be useful to individuals with MS.

One of the main components of the Ticket to Work program deals with consumer choice. When an individual receives a Ticket to Work in the mail, he or she can elect to use it or not. This is a voluntary program, so there is no requirement for the ticket-holder to use the ticket. If the ticket holder chooses to use it, the SSA assigns the ticket to an Employment Network (EN). ENs consist of agencies, organizations, or individuals that have gone through SSA's approval process and can provide vocational rehabilitation services. Prior to the Ticket to Work program, an individual would automatically be referred to a local state vocational rehabilitation (VR) agency. The Ticket to Work program offers the individual greater choice—he or she can still receive support services and assistance from a state VR agency or from any other EN of his or her choice. A directory of Employment Networks can be found at www.yourtickettowork.com or by calling 1-866-968-7842.

Once the Social Security disability recipient determines which Employment Network to work with, the ticket is assigned to that network. Vocational services and supports vary from EN to EN, so the Ticket to Work recipients must do research to find a network that will provide them with the services they anticipate requiring in order to return to work.

Another program that was created under TWWIIA that can be very useful to Social Security disability recipients is the Benefits Planning Assistance and Outreach (BPAO) program, later renamed the Work Incentives Planning and Assistance (WIPA) program. WIPA programs exist in every community and provide free benefits planning and counseling to Social Security recipients. Trained staff members work with people to determine the impact that work would have on their benefits. This allows individuals to learn more about all the work incentives available to protect their benefits (including those described earlier in this chapter). The key is to be as informed and educated as possible. By being knowledgeable of the impact that work would have on benefits, including other benefit programs like food stamps and Section 8 housing, the individual can make an informed choice and realistically decide if returning to work is in his or her best interest. According to the SSA's Work Site (14), a WIPA program can do the following:

- Answer your questions about how part-time, full-time, or seasonal work would affect your individual disability benefits and other benefits you may receive from federal, state, and local programs.
- Answer your questions about how work would affect your health care.
- Answer your questions about SSA work incentives and work incentives of other programs.
- Discuss your individual employment goals, including possible barriers and the resources or services you would need to overcome any barriers. A WIPA can also help you find those resources and services.
- Help you plan how to use work incentives or other benefits for a successful return to work.
- Help you work with your local Social Security office to put in place the work incentives that you need.
- Help you use your Ticket to Work and find an Employment Network that is right for you.

Other useful components of TWWIIA deal with continuation of medical insurance benefits and expedited reinstatement of benefits. TWWIIA extended Medicare coverage up to 8.5 years after Social Security benefits have stopped. This includes premium-free Part A coverage as well as Part B for the annual premium. Some states also allow a Medicaid buy-in. In addition, once benefits have ceased due to earnings from work, if a person becomes unable to work again because of a medical condition, her or she can request that his or her benefits be reinstated without having to file a new application. The benefits would include the financial benefit, as well as Medicare and Medicaid, depending on what insurance benefit the individual was receiving. The person must make that request within 60 months from the month that his or her benefits were terminated.

Incentives versus Disincentives

Even though work incentives are available and the Ticket to Work program provides ways to deal with concerns over losing health insurance benefits and getting reinstated for benefits quickly if a person's disease changes over time, there are still inherent disincentives in the Social Security program for individuals with MS. Oftentimes, the person with MS may prefer to utilize the work incentives as a means to supplement or complement their disability income. Given the unpredictability of the disease, the variability of symptoms from time to time, and the overall progressive nature of MS, the person may be concerned about losing the benefits altogether. Instead, he or she may rather work within the guidelines of the work incentive and retain benefits while possibly working part-time. This strategy would serve to protect one's Social Security benefits, but it also relegates the beneficiary to part-time employment and a fixed income as long as he or she is beholden to Social Security income and asset restrictions. Indeed, numerous surveys over the past several decades regarding the employment concerns of people with MS have found work disincentives in the SSA programs, both real and perceived, among the most frequently cited reasons for the high rate of unemployment among people with MS (15).

Summary

Generally speaking, people are better off working than not working, even as they cope with MS, but for some people the onset and progression of MS combine with other life circumstances to make continued employment infeasible or impossible. For those people with MS who decide to leave the work force, help may be available from the SSA in the form of cash monthly allowances or health insurance coverage.

Supplemental Security Income (SSI) is available to people with disabilities who are too disabled to work and who have limited financial resources and limited recent work histories. Funded by general income tax contributions in partnership with states, SSI payments can be accompanied by health insurance coverage from Medicaid. Social Security Disability Insurance (SSDI) is for people with disabilities who are too disabled to work and who have substantial recent work histories. Funded by FICA taxes specifically earmarked for Social Security, SSDI constitutes America's only nationalized disability insurance program. SSDI payments are often accompanied by health insurance coverage from Medicare.

Although SSI and SSDI benefits are only available to people who are not able to perform substantial gainful employment because of their disabilities, the SSA does offer a number of work incentives designed to encourage SSI and SSDI beneficiaries to enter or reenter the work force and thus eliminate the need for Social Security benefits. Even so, many people with MS cite disincentives in SSI and SSDI as some of the main reasons they do not continue working until retirement age. There is a "catch 22" inherent in the SSA's policies whereby people cannot receive

146

SSI or SSDI benefits unless they are too disabled to work, but if they become able to work again, they stand to lose their benefits. The threat of losing their benefits often dissuade people from resuming their careers once SSI or SSDI has taken effect, which often leaves people with MS or other disabilities no other choice but to persist in unemployment until retirement age; therefore, we believe that SSI and SSDI benefits should be viewed as a "last resort" after all other options to continue working have been exhausted.

By understanding Social Security's rules and regulations regarding documentation of disability, application processes, appeals and reconsiderations, work incentives, and the limitations of SSI and SSDI benefits, people with MS will be able to make the best choice regarding whether and when to discontinue their employment. Becoming knowledgeable about SSI and SSDI will also ensure that individuals secure the maximum level of benefits for which they are eligible.

References

1. Social Security Administration (2007, May). *What we mean by disability.* Retrieved May 28, 2007, from Social Security Online: www.ssa.gov/dibplan/ dqualify4.htm.
2. Social Security Administration (2006, June). *Disability evaluation under Social Security.* Retrieved May 28, 2007, from Social Security Online: www.ssa.gov/disability/professionals/bluebook/.
3. Social Security Administration (2006). *The Blue Book: Disability evaluation under Social Security.* Washington, DC: Author.
4. Social Security Administration (2005, January). *What we mean by disability: neurological adult.* Retrieved May 28, 2007, from Social Security Online: www.ssa.gov/disability/professionals/bluebook/11.00-Neurological-Adult.htm#11.09%20Multiple%20sclerosis.
5. Social Security Administration (2007, July). *Supplemental security income.* Retrieved May 28, 2007, from Social Security Online: www.ssa.gov/notices/supplemental-security-income/.
6. Social Security Administration (2007, February). *How much work do you need?* Retrieved May 28, 2007, from Social Security Online: www.ssa.gov/dibplan/dqualify2.htm.
7. Northrop, D., Cooper, S., & Calder, K. (2007). Health insurance resources: Options for people with chronic disease or disability. New York: Demos Medical Publishing, p. 42.
8. Social Security Administration (2007, January). *Federal review process.* Retrieved June 16, 2007, from Social Security Online: www.socialsecurity.gov/appeals/court_process.html.
9. The Henry J. Kaiser Family Foundation (2003, January). *Kaiser Commission on Medicaid and the uninsured.* Retrieved July 15, 2007 from kff.org: www.kff.org/medicaid/2236-index.cfm.
10. U.S. Department of Health and Human Services (2007, January). My *Medicare enrollment.* Retrieved July 15, 2007, from MyMedicare.gov: www.medicare.gov/ MedicareEligibility/home.asp?version=default&browser= IE%7C6%7CWinXP&language=English.

11. U.S. Department of Health and Human Services (2007, August). *Medicare spotlights.* Retrieved May 28, 2007, from MyMedicare.gov: www.medicare.gov.

12. Social Security Administration (2007). *2007 Red Book.* Retrieved May 28, 2007, from Social Security Online: www.socialsecurity.gov/redbook/eng/main.htm.

13. Hennessey, M., & Rumrill, P. (2007). Key employment concerns for people with multiple sclerosis. In R. Kalb (Ed.), *Multiple sclerosis: The questions you have, the answers you need.* New York: Demos Medical Publishing, p 320.

14. Social Security Administration (2007, August). *Work incentives planning and assistance cooperative agreement awards.* Retrieved May 28, 2007, from Social Security Online: www.socialsecurity.gov/work/ServiceProviders/WIPADirectory.html.

15. Rumrill, P., & Hennessey, M. (2001). *Multiple sclerosis: A guide for health care and rehabilitation professionals.* Springfield, IL: Charles C Thomas.

8 An Employment Perspective From The National Multiple Sclerosis Society

Steven W. Nissen

MULTIPLE SCLEROSIS (MS) stops people from moving. The National Multiple Sclerosis Society (NMSS) exists to make sure it doesn't. It addresses the challenges of each person affected by MS by funding cutting edge research, driving change through advocacy, facilitating professional education, collaborating with MS organizations around the world, and providing programs and services designed to help people with MS and their families move their lives forward. Founded in 1946 by Sylvia Lawry, the NMSS's home office and 50-state network of chapters devoted over $125 million in 2006 to programs that enhanced people's lives and also invested over $46 million to support 380 research projects around the world. We want to do something about MS NOW, and are dedicated to achieving a world free of MS. Join the movement at www.nationalMSsociety.org or by calling 1-800-344-4867.

Employment plays an integral part in our lives. People work for a variety of reasons including the obvious benefits such as a paycheck, health and retirement benefits, and financial security. But work, often-times, is about more than the bottom line. It relates to self-esteem, self-worth, feelings of contributing to society, and being part of a larger organization or company. When MS enters the picture, it has the potential of throwing a person's life into upheaval, including his or her employment situation. We know from the research that the majority of people with MS who had been working leave the work force prematurely and voluntarily. People with MS have a higher rate of unemployment when compared to those with other chronic illnesses or disabilities. The NMSS has had to address employment issues consciously and proactively. The NMSS has long been involved in employment-related research; has developed tools, training programs, and publications that chapter staff can utilize when working with individuals with MS and with employers; set forth the minimum standards for employment programs to be offered at the chapter level and minimum level of employment knowledge that chapter staff members should have; and offered specific tools for the employer community. These efforts were intensified after the passage of the Americans with Disabilities Act (ADA) in 1990.

12 Guiding Principles

In 1991, the NMSS reaffirmed its commitment to support the employment efforts of people with MS. Twelve guiding principles were originally proposed in a position paper entitled "Employment Issues in Multiple Sclerosis." Those principles are:

1. Disability in itself should never be assumed to reduce the capability of an individual to work.
2. The Society supports the concepts and principles of the ADA and commits to taking a lead role in its implementation.
3. Barrier-free and accessible environments are crucial to maximize employment opportunities for people with disabilities.
4. Small accommodations in the work environment can enable many citizens with disabilities to be productively employed.
5. Negative attitudes toward people with disabilities create a major barrier to their employment. Responsibility for changing attitudes must be shared by business, government, public and private sector agencies, health care providers, the media, labor, educators, and people with disabilities themselves.
6. The Society supports legislative change to remove work disincentives for those with disabilities and advocates implementation of policies to help people with disabilities access their rights under the law.
7. The Society supports legislation that provides incentives to employers to promote the employment of people with disabilities.

8. The Society urges changes in vocational rehabilitation policies that facilitate the employment of people with MS.
9. The Society supports research to benefit those with MS and other disabilities by promoting understanding of work-related issues and identifying solutions to existing problems. This includes the continuing development of technology that will enable people with disabilities to perform more jobs. Such technology should be made available and affordable.
10. The Society supports the development of a comprehensive long-term care system that provides social, health, and personal services for all Americans.
11. The Society applauds businesses and organizations that have voluntary plans for significant and special efforts (affirmative action) in the recruitment and accommodation of employees with disabilities.
12. Programs and policies that are intended to assist people with disabilities should reflect the opinions of those whose lives will be affected by their practices.

These principles continue to be relevant today.

Program Planning and Analysis Guide (2003 to 2007)

The NMSS, through its Program Planning and Analysis Guidelines (PPAG), had set forth the core nationwide requirements and elective activities that chapters were to provide. The overall goal related to employment was to "help people with MS to maintain and enhance employment and to explore career options" (1, p. 8). Activities that chapters were expected to provide or could elect to provide included the following (1):

Nationwide Core Programs and Activities

1. Maintain information on issues and services related to employment (e.g., the *Technical Assistance Manual* of Title I of the ADA, Social Security work incentives, Job Accommodation Network, temporary employment agencies, career counseling, assistive technology).
2. All chapter information and referral providers can discuss basic employment issues (referrals to vocational rehabilitation, information in NMSS brochures on employment).
3. The chapter provides access to consultation on complex employment issues (e.g., continuing to work versus leaving the work force, disclosing, requesting reasonable accommodations, understanding disability

benefits, and staying aware of legislation pertinent to employment, such as the expanded Social Security Work Incentives, Title I of the ADA). *Note:* To accomplish this goal, the chapter should have a staff member trained as an employment advisor who can discuss all aspects of employment. The MS Employment Advisor Training course will prepare the designated staff member to become an employment advisor. A chapter may collaborate and share an agreement with a community expert to provide employment consultation. A chapter may contract with the Kent State University Career Counseling Service for the client.

4. Develop and maintain relationships with key staff members of state vocational rehabilitation (VR) agencies.

Elective Programs

1. Conduct/collaborate on an education program or in-service on MS for state vocational rehabilitation staff, private vocational rehabilitation agencies, Veteran's Administration personnel, and/or employment/career counselors.
2. Provide an education program on maintaining employment (e.g., teleconference series, group program). This program can be a component or track in a large elective educational program.
3. Educate and/or network with employers and/or employment specialists and employees by doing any of the following:

    - Promote a local job fair to clients.
    - Develop a business advisory committee to assist the chapter in delivery of employment programs.
    - Engage select employers and local entrepreneurs in mock job interviews for people with MS seeking career changes, in coaching, or in helping people with MS explore traditional and nontraditional career options.
    - Develop an innovative approach to educating and/or networking with employers.
    - Submit a nomination for the NMSS employer of the year award and recognize this employer locally.

4. Conduct/cosponsor program for employers that may lead to increased employment of people with disabilities (e.g., provide speaker for corporate employee attitudinal training program or

disability awareness day, or for professional group such as American Society of Training and Development or Society of Human Resource Professionals).

5. Work collaboratively with a local employment agency that specializes in placement of people with disabilities (e.g., state or community agency, temporary employment agency, job service).

6. Provide a specialized series program that helps people work through career options and decisions (e.g., national video program on working with MS).

7. Offer original program designed to achieve employment goals. Determine and measure outcomes.

These activities speak to the minimum level of employment-related knowledge required by chapters, and challenge chapter staff to offer programs.

There were several lessons learned from requiring that the employment PPAG be implemented. Oftentimes, chapter staff members were fearful and apprehensive of addressing employment issues and concerns. Staff members were often handling varied concerns of individuals affected by MS and planning a variety of programs. Employment was one more thing added to that person's job description. Many felt compelled to try to find jobs for people with MS even though job placement was not a service that chapters were expected to offer. To provide chapters the tools needed to alleviate pressures on staff members, the NMSS designed the Employment and MS Advisor training described later in this chapter.

Quality of Life Principles

In 2007, the NMSS replaced the PPAG with the Multiple Sclerosis International Federation's (MSIF) Quality of Life (QOL) principles. Understanding that MS can affect a person's quality of life,

it is important to work to maintain or improve QOL for people with MS, utilizing a broad range of approaches such as those described in these principles. The development of the principles was based on a series of interviews, a literature review, the clinical, programmatic, and research experience of the authors, and review by a Work Group and technical Oversight Group organized by the Multiple Sclerosis International Federation (MSIF) (2, p. 17).

The 10 Quality of Life principles include the following:

- Independence and empowerment
- Medical care
- Continuing (long-term or social) care
- Health promotion and disease prevention
- Support for family members
- Transportation
- Employment and volunteer activities
- Disability benefits and cash assistance
- Education
- Housing and accessibility of buildings in the community

As it relates to the employment quality of life principle, the overall goal is that "Support systems and services are available to enable people with MS to continue employment as long as they are productive and desire to work" (2, p. 33).

The Principles to Promote the Quality of Life of People with Multiple Sclerosis (2, 33–34) states the following:

Many people with MS leave the [labor] force because of the symptoms of the disease, such as fatigue, functional disability, and cognitive impairment. Leaving the workforce can have a major effect on family income as well as an individual's [self-esteem]. Some people with MS could continue to work if employers provide assistance and restructure their work. A wide range of accommodations or adaptations are possible, including part-time work, additional breaks in the work day, working only mornings, reducing the room temperature, changing work tasks, telecommuting, reducing travel, providing ramps, providing offices near restrooms, and others. Governments and social service providers can contribute by providing vocational rehabilitation and training programmes. For those people with MS who do leave the [labor] force, substitute activities are important to sustain a sense of purpose in life. Examples include voluntary activities, creative arts, serving as MS peer counsellors, assisting with MS Society or MS centre administration or advocacy efforts, pursuing further education, and others.

These statements summarize the important tenets of the NMSS. People with MS should be encouraged to work as long as they choose to but often leave due to challenging symptoms. The impact of leaving the workplace is far reaching and can affect a person's sense of self. Accommodations can prove beneficial for people with MS, and there should be support services in place, including vocational rehabilitation services.

Another key tenet of the Quality of Life Principles is to assess the needs of unique communities. Whereas the PPAG employment category offered "standardized" activities and programs, the QOL suggests that chapters look at the specific needs of the individuals and communities they are serving. This allows for much more creativity in how employment issues are addressed, the types of programs that are offered, and the proposed outcomes of those initiatives.

Programs, Publications, Training Initiatives, and Research Initiatives

Since the guiding principles were initially set forth, and in support of PPAG requirements and Quality of Life Principles, the NMSS has offered a variety of employment programs and initiatives designed to achieve successful employment outcomes for people with MS. These include Operation Job Match, Job Raising, Project Alliance, Career Crossroads: Employment and MS, MS in the Workplace: A Guide for Employers (see Chapter 4), and grants from federal and private agencies. Joyce Nelson, President and Chief Executive Officer of the NMSS, states that

> Data from our Sonya Slifka Longitudinal Study show that even with better treatments and workplace changes, 56% of people with MS are still unemployed. Our programs and services help people to explore their options for continued employment—even when career changes are necessary to accommodate MS symptoms.

This clearly shows the importance placed on employment programs, including Career Crossroads: Employment and MS, and other services intended to improve these figures. There are several publications and manuals available for individuals with MS, employers, and chapter staff and volunteers.

Publications for the Employer Community and Individuals with MS

The NMSS recognizes the importance of addressing employment and has a variety of materials available. Publications available from local chapters, written primarily for individuals with MS, include titles such as *The Win-Win Approach to Reasonable Accommodations, ADA and People with MS, A Place in the Workplace, Should I Work?*, and *Disclosure: The Basic Facts*. For employers, the NMSS offers a publication entitled *Information for Employers*, as well as the DVD, *MS in the Workplace: A Guide for Employers*, which were previously described in Chapter 4.

KNOWLEDGE IS POWER—INFORMATION FOR INDIVIDUALS NEWLY DIAGNOSED WITH MS. Knowledge is Power is an at-home education program for the newly diagnosed person with MS. This 6-week program allows individuals to receive educational materials via postal mail or e-mail. Topics covered in this program include:

- Taking the First Steps: What is MS? Dealing with Your Diagnosis & Disclosure
- Disease-modifying Treatments for MS
- Maximizing Your Employment Options
- Treating Yourself Well
- Maintaining Healthy Relationships: Family, Friends, and Colleagues
- Working with Your Doctor

Employment information is an important part of this program. It is imperative that newly diagnosed persons be aware of the impact that MS can have on employment, learn how to handle the challenges, and identify sources to turn to for assistance, including the NMSS.

EMPLOYMENT PROGRAMS MANUAL. To assist chapter staff in addressing employment goals and activities, the NMSS has several manuals and training resources available for chapter staff. The *Employment Programs Manual* (1) provides guidelines and resources that chapters can use to plan, develop, and implement client programs to help people with MS maintain and enhance their employment and explore career options. Included in this manual are seven sections:

- Introduction including background and rationale for including employment programs
- Summarizing the Program Planning and Analysis Guidelines pertaining to the employment goal

- Program development including definition of the goals and objectives of employment programs, format ideas, speaker suggestions, statement of staff and volunteer roles, and curriculum suggestions
- Program implementation including ways to promote employment programs, collaborate with other organizations, and evaluate program outcomes
- Resources including contact information for employment and/or disability-related agencies and organizations, and Internet resources
- Listing of employment-related NMSS publications
- Checklist chapter staff can use to help plan and implement employment programs.

Information in this manual can be utilized by the chapters to offer relevant and important programs to address the employment needs of the individuals they serve.

EMPLOYERS MANUAL. *Providing Information About MS to Employers* (3) is available to assist chapter staff in educating the employer community about MS and the advantages of hiring and retaining employees with MS. Included are formats that can be used for employer programs, ways to locate potential speakers, tips for conducting an employer visit, and a sample presentation outline. General disability awareness information is provided to dispel some of the myths about people with disabilities in the workplace, to recommend disability-friendly strategies, to provide general information about employer responsibilities under the ADA, about other pertinent legislation that may pertain to someone with MS, and about tax incentives for employers who hire and accommodate people with disabilities. Specific practical accommodation strategies are outlined. The more common symptoms of MS and ways those symptoms can be accommodated are given. Extensive resources including publications, agencies, and Internet websites are listed. Portions of the information contained in this manual can also be utilized by NMSS staff in conducting in-service trainings for vocational rehabilitation counselors.

VOCATIONAL EDUCATION FOR NMSS STAFF WORKING WITH PEOPLE WITH MS. Beginning in 2001, the NMSS expanded its training to include Employment and MS training for chapter staff and key volunteers. As stated above in the discussion of the PPAG, the expectation was that in each NMSS chapter someone would act as the employment advisor—screening employment calls, doing a comprehensive assessment, providing relevant and accurate employment information, and making appropriate referrals to other agencies. This employment advisor was often a chapter staff member. Some chapters have agreements with a key volunteer with a background in vocational rehabilitation to whom the chapter can refer the individual for more intensive employment assistance. The Employment and MS training was designed to provide the baseline level of knowledge related to employment issues. For a chapter that does not have a vocational rehabilitation counselor on staff, the Employment and MS training can help existent staff to be well informed in their response to employment queries. The Employment and MS training provides information on the following topics:

- The employment continuum
- Disclosure and accommodations
- Legal protections—ADA, Family and Medical Leave Act, Health Insurance Portability and Accountability Act, and Consolidated Omnibus Budget Reconciliation Act
- How to handle employment discrimination—where to refer the person who is inquiring
- Private short-term and long-term disability as well as federal disability insurance options—Social Security Administration administered benefits
- The federal disability benefit process and work incentives
- Resources and referrals including the state vocational rehabilitation agency and the Job Accommodation Network
- Sample forms and checklists that could be used, including a sample of the form used to refer someone to the state vocational rehabilitation agency and the Social Security Administration's guidelines used in determining disability for a person with MS

The Employment and MS training is comprised of five modules. Each participant is assigned an employment coach, someone contracted by the national office to work with the individual participant in bringing the training to life, discussing real-life issues that come up, and challenging the participant. Coaches are either current or former staff members drawn from several chapters of the NMSS. Throughout the training, participants are encouraged to complete homework activities and to keep a journal of calls they have taken on employment issues. At the conclusion of each module, there is a quiz that is reviewed with the coach. Once the coach feels the participant has successfully completed the course, a completion certificate is sent to the individual.

In taking a closer look at the topics covered in this training, it is important to note that information is provided about issues that may present themselves at any time throughout the entire continuum of employment. Individuals with MS may have left the workplace or be trying to decide if they should leave. It is important to be familiar with disability options, work incentives, and work disincentives. The individual with MS may not have explored all of the employment options prior to separating from the workplace and needs to know that he or she can turn to the NMSS to address these issues, as well.

The Employment and MS training is designed to give chapter staff the tools they need to appropriately and effectively handle the employment calls, and be prepared and confident in addressing employment issues. Persons with MS can turn to the NMSS for answers to their employment questions and in so doing feel more confident making employment decisions before being faced with an employment crisis.

RESEARCH INITIATIVES. The NMSS's Research and Clinical Programs department has funded several employment-related projects and research studies designed to better understand the employment concerns and barriers facing individuals with MS. Dr. Nicholas LaRocca, Associate Vice President for Health Care Delivery and Policy Research, states,

> The employment picture for people with MS has improved over the years due to changes such as the ADA and better awareness. However, we face continuing challenges, particularly how best to address cognitive changes and lingering examples of discrimination. So we need to redouble our efforts to address employment among people with MS through research, advocacy, and programs.

The NMSS has recognized the importance of funding employment-related research and will continue to do so in the future.

Looking Toward the Future

Neurologists, other health care providers, and family members and friends are advised to stop prescribing unemployment as a course of treatment for people with MS. Doctors and other well-meaning individuals may suggest that the person with MS leave the workplace because they believe work is too stressful and could exacerbate the disease. This is not accurate. Unemployment does not cure stress—in fact, unemployment may lead to additional stress caused by reducing income, resulting in the loss of health insurance benefits, and creating financial and household instability.

Oftentimes, the individuals with MS do not contact their chapter until they (a) are in a time of crisis, (b) are at risk for losing the job, (c) have had a negative performance evaluation that could have been prevented had accommodations been implemented, (d) have been wrongfully terminated once the MS was disclosed to the employer, and/or (e) experience poor performance at work but have not disclosed to anyone for fear of being seen as different. Nancy Law, Executive Vice President of Programs and Services, states,

> Some of our most important program initiatives focus on helping people in their first years after diagnosis. The time to think about how MS will fit into your career and your life is not when you are struggling to keep up at work or about to lose your job. Make career planning a priority right from the start.

This comment clearly addresses the need to be proactive in regard to employment, plan ahead, and discuss employment issues BEFORE being faced with a crisis.

We have had to address these issues creatively and proactively by ensuring that the individuals we serve feel confident turning to the NMSS to address their employment fears, questions, and concerns. We have materials and trainings available to chapter staff, employment-related publications available for individuals with MS and employers, and programs available directly to our constituents. Ms. Law says,

> We are seeing people newly diagnosed with MS staying in the workplace longer. Many employers do understand their obligations for reasonable accommodations, and are not only willing

but eager to do what they can to keep valued employees. And certainly improvements in the treatment and management of MS have made a difference.

We will continue to do all that we can to guide and support persons with MS in their decisions about employment.

References

1. National Multiple Sclerosis Society (2005). *Employment programs manual.* Denver: National Multiple Sclerosis Society Programs and Services Department.
2. MSIF (2005). *Principles to promote the quality of life of people with multiple sclerosis.* London: Multiple Sclerosis International Federation (MSIF). Downloadable at www.msif.org/en/publications/quality_of_life_principles/index.html.
3. National Multiple Sclerosis Society (2005). *Providing information about MS to employers.* Denver: National Multiple Sclerosis Society Programs and Services Department.

Policy, Programming, and Research Recommendations to Improve the Employment Prospects of People with Multiple Sclerosis

Phillip D. Rumrill, Jr.

THIS BOOK REFLECTS THE considerable compendium of research that has been devoted to the employment implications of multiple sclerosis (MS). As advancements in treatment, symptom management, vocational assessment strategies, placement and retention programs, and federal legislation continue to hold significant promise for members of the MS community and their families and friends, the troubling fact remains that far too few people with MS are presently engaged in the labor force.

Unfortunately, this underrepresentation is occurring at a time when employers need well-trained, experienced workers more than they have at any point in recent history. According to Mullins et al. (1), the ever-aging American populace (a function of the "baby boom" generation having fewer children than its parents had and longer life expectancies) will have decreasing numbers of working-age constituents from which to draw over the next three decades. Therefore, they exhorted the rehabilitation profession and the employer community to work together to identify strategies to place, accommodate, and maintain qualified people with disabilities in work roles. Several facts make people with MS an ideal labor pool for employers seeking to meet society's growing need for diversity in the workplace:

1. The vast majority (more than 90 percent) of people with MS have employment histories (2,3).
2. The onset of the illness typically occurs at around age 30—usually after the individual has established a career (4).
3. People with MS are well-educated; 97 percent are high school graduates and 40 percent are college graduates (5).
4. Employers report that most workers with MS perform at levels equal to or higher than nondisabled employees (6).
5. More than half of the accommodations used by employees with MS cost nothing or very little (under $50) to implement (3,7).

It should be noted that people with MS are not unique among members of the disability community in their ability to succeed in employment. According to the DuPont Corporation (8, p.3.), among people with disabilities, "[employers] will find a pool of qualified, motivated employees." As early as 1954, for example, long before enactment of the Rehabilitation Act and the Americans with Disabilities Act, a survey of New York City businesses found the performance of employees with disabilities equal to the performance of nondisabled workers (9). In fact, one-third of employers in that survey rated employees with disabilities as superior workers. In a 1961 study, more than 60 percent of managers and supervisors reported that employees with disabilities were more conscientious about their work and more independent than their nondisabled colleagues (10).

More recently, findings from DuPont's (8) 40-year study of workers with disabilities support the company's prediction that Americans with disabilities will provide a valuable resource for twenty-first century employers. Over the past four decades, 97 percent of DuPont's employees with disabilities were rated average or above in safety. In attendance, 86 percent were rated average or above. In overall job performance, some 90 percent received average or above average ratings. Significantly, these impressive evaluations have not been limited to employees in entry-level or unskilled occupations; nearly half (45 percent) of DuPont's 1990 employees with disabilities held technical, managerial, or professional positions (8).

Indeed, people with MS who keep their jobs have proven equal to the task in the workplace. Why, then, do so many leave their jobs, often before the occurrence of severe symptoms? To the extent that researchers have found limited success to date in explaining the high rate of unemployment among people with MS, a more applied, problem-solving focus is warranted.

Specifically, this chapter attempts to answer the question, What can researchers, practitioners, policy makers, employers, disability advocates, and people with MS themselves do to increase the rate of labor force participation within the American MS community?

Recommendation 1: Continue the Search for a Cure and Increasingly Effective Treatments

Although the severity of medical symptoms does not completely determine whether a person with MS will acquire or maintain employment, efforts to minimize or eliminate the effects of the illness can only aid the rehabilitation process. The search for preventative and arrestive cures has been hampered by the elusiveness of the disease's origin (scientists have been unable to determine with certainty how a person develops MS), but recent treatments such as those described in Chapter 1 have shown some promise in alleviating the far-reaching psychomedical impact of the illness (4).

Illness and disability prevention initiatives have not always met with unanimous favor among disability groups. In *No Pity*, an excellent historical account of the "disability rights" movement in the United States, Shapiro (11) noted that many disability advocates oppose medical research that seeks to cure existing disabling conditions. The argument against such measures is that they degrade and dehumanize people who already have those conditions, and that they could deprive people of the opportunity to have a disability. Certain groups have gone so far as to challenge mandatory seat belt and lower speed limit laws (which decrease spinal cord and traumatic brain injuries), early prenatal screenings for potential birth defects, and cochlear implants for people who are deaf, suggesting that these measures stand to reduce the constituency and consequent strength of the disability community.

This author does not share these views. Multiple sclerosis research directed at finding a cure and refining treatments must continue. Efforts to prevent or treat disabilities do not preclude acceptance of people who have those disabilities, and I believe that most people with MS— even those who have effectively adjusted to the illness—would prefer not to have developed the disease in the first place. Hence, people's prospects for increased independence, the abiding mission of both the disability rights movement and the vocational rehabilitation process, will be enhanced, not hindered, by future medical advancements in MS research.

Recommendation 2: Target Members of Traditionally Underserved Populations who have MS

To the extent that minority status presents an inherent disadvantage in the career development process in the general population (12), it seems logical that coupling MS with membership in a traditionally underserved group could pose a "double obstacle" to employment success. It has been documented that women, who comprise a decided majority of the American MS community, find it more difficult to maintain employment while coping with the illness than do men (13). Also experiencing particular difficulty are people with MS whose occupations require less education and demand significant physical exertion (14). Accordingly, special effort should be made to direct employment initiatives such as those described in Chapter 4 toward those people with MS who need them the most. In addition to women and people with lower educational attainment, these "high-need" groups may include people of color (although the worldwide MS population is predominantly white), individuals who reside in rural areas, and people who do not have successful employment histories.

Recommendation 3: Focus on Success: What Factors Enable People with MS to Keep their Jobs?

The majority of research on the employment of people with disabilities focuses on the difficulties that people encounter in every stage of the career development process. Even in this book, much of the focus has been placed on such negative aspects of the world of work as unemployment, on-the-job barriers, functional decrements, workplace discrimination, and psychological problems. What about the people with MS who successfully maintain employment? What can researchers, practitioners, and people with MS learn from them to help those who are confronted with the difficulties noted here? People with MS comprise a qualified, capable, and seasoned labor resource, and people seeking to actualize their talents can learn a great deal from their community leaders, support group members, and friends who have MS, and who have successfully negotiated the rigors and uncertainty of working with an unpredictable, chronic illness. Critical incident analyses from the qualitative research paradigm (15) provide a mechanism for reporting case studies of successfully employed people with MS, the factors that led to their success, and the resources they marshaled in pursuit of their career goals.

Recommendation 4: Encourage Utilization of Vocational Rehabilitation Services

The fact that people with MS underutilize vocational rehabilitation services does not mean that they are disproportionably ineligible for those services. Even people with MS whose disabilities are not "severe" enough to render them eligible for paid services can receive valuable personal consultation and referral services from vocational rehabilitation agencies. Physicians, nurses, social workers, and other service providers must refer their patients and clients with MS (especially those dealing with the most severe symptoms) to the vocational rehabilitation program as a matter of course. Most vocational rehabilitation agencies operate under an "order of selection" (16) mandate whereby services are prioritized in favor of people with the most severe disabilities when applying for vocational rehabilitation services; it is therefore, essential for people with MS to provide the fullest possible accounts of the ways and life areas in which MS effects them.

Recommendation 5: Develop Early Intervention Strategies to Help People with MS Keep their Jobs

To the extent that the most precipitous decline in physical functioning typically occurs during the first 5 years after diagnosis of MS (4), recently diagnosed people (the majority of whom are employed) may need assistance with such on-the-job issues as knowing when and how to disclose any disability-related work limitations, identifying how those limitations could be overcome via reasonable accommodations, and requesting accommodations from their employers as per Title I of the Americans with Disability Act (ADA) (3,7). Unfortunately, these pressing needs for employment assistance occur at a time when a considerable portion of the person's energy is being devoted to psychological adjustment to the disease itself (4), reassessment of other social roles, learning more about the disease, and symptom management. With all of these considerations, it is understandable that employment may not be the person's most prominent concern during the early stages of MS. However, because career identity constitutes a defining attribute for many people (what one does for work is who one is), the issue of work must be addressed as part of the person's medical, personal, and social orientation to MS.

Specifically, health care professionals, social workers, psychologists, and rehabilitation professionals must work closely with consumer advocacy groups to provide coordinated, early-intervention support for people with MS, support that is offered within a job retention and career maintenance context. Many chapters of the National Multiple Sclerosis Society offer "newly diagnosed" support groups, and the vocational implications of MS should be systematically addressed in those programs. Finally, I wish to implore physicians to refrain from prescribing unemployment as a treatment strategy. The therapeutic benefits of working (not to mention the potentially devastating psychological impact of not working) make it imperative for responsible practitioners to encourage anyone who wants to work to continue to do so. If and when the person with MS chooses to stop working, that decision must be that person's alone. Of course, career-related decisions should and do incorporate advice and guidance from significant others and health care and rehabilitation professionals, but this critically important decision must be finalized by the affected person.

Recommendation 6: Provide Ongoing Employment Assistance: Early Interventions are Necessary but not Sufficient

The difficulties associated with maintaining employment while coping with disability are by no means unique to people with MS. In fact, studies show that people with disabilities in general need more support in the job retention process than is presently available within existing service delivery mechanisms.

Roessler and Bolton (17) documented a "lateral movement phenomenon" in their follow-up survey of 57 former vocational rehabilitation clients with various disabilities. Career patterns of respondents consisted primarily of changes from one entry-level job to another, often interspersed with extended periods of unemployment (18) also substantiated the problems that people with disabilities have in holding jobs following initial placement. Their study of 66 people with disabilities who had completed a postsecondary transition program revealed an encouraging 68 percent employment rate at a 1-year follow-up. However, 36 percent of those participants who were employed had not been continuously employed for the entire 1-year period. Moreover, participants' occupational changes during the follow-up period tended to follow Roessler and Bolton's (17) lateral pattern.

Perhaps the most compelling rationale for increased postemployment services for people with disabilities can be drawn from data reported by Gibbs (19). In a follow-up survey of 2,536 former vocational rehabilitation clients whose cases had been closed by virtue of successful employment, Gibbs found initial periods of employment of less than 3 months among some 25 percent of respondents. One year after case closure, only 51 percent were still employed. During Gibb's 54-month tracking period, no less than 84.4 percent of these successful rehabilitants experienced some interruption of employment, and many were never reemployed.

Indeed, although the vocational rehabilitation program (the nation's oldest and largest service system for people with disabilities) purports to "rehabilitate" more than half of its clients, it appears to have a short-term (at best) impact on clients' abilities to work and live independently. Two years after "successful" case closure, rehabilitants' mean income drops below the income that they reported at the time of enrollment in the vocational rehabilitation program (20).

From these findings, it should be clear that people with MS are not alone in their need for effective and comprehensive postemployment services. However, the unpredictable, often episodic nature of the illness does warrant special consideration on the part of employees, employers, and service providers alike. On-the-job interventions that address the employee's unique and often fluctuating needs must be available on an ongoing, as-needed basis if the person with MS is to maintain and fully succeed in his or her career.

Recommendation 7: Encourage Self-Advocacy and Consumer Involvement

With the fairly recent enactment of the ADA and a growing societal commitment to include people with disabilities in every aspect of life, people with MS and other disabilities are being expected to take a more active role in society than ever before. As mainstream structures and institutions continue to reduce the barriers to inclusion, active involvement stands to become less of a concession to people with disabilities and more of a requirement for them. The provisions of the ADA, for example, call for a great deal of initiative on the part of individuals with disabilities in asserting their civil rights to accessible employment opportunities, public services, public accommodations, and communication systems.

With respect to employment, Title I of the ADA (see Chapter 5) requires people with a disability to take an active role in (a) requesting reasonable accommodations from their employer, (b) identifying resources that can facilitate the accommodation process, and (c) monitoring the ongoing effectiveness of on-the-job accommodations (21). It also requires those who have experienced employment discrimination to file a formal complaint and follow a series of administrative and legal procedures. Hence, people with MS need accurate information about their rights under the ADA. They may also require individual or group consultation concerning the often complicated nuances of civil rights law and how to access the protections to which they are entitled.

Recommendation 8: Make Employment a Priority: No One is "Too Disabled" to Work

Some experts have suggested that the woeful rate of labor force participation among Americans with disabilities is attributable in part to the fact that society "excuses" people whom it considers unable to work (22). However, the idea of a person being "too disabled" to work has come under fire recently. Research indicates that the severity of a person's disability has little bearing on his or her prospects for successful rehabilitation; rather, such factors as motivation and residual abilities are more predictive of success (23,24). Accordingly, many contemporary job placement and retention programs are predicated on the assumption that anyone who wants to work can work and should be encouraged to do so to every extent possible—regardless of disability (25).

To make employment a viable option for people diagnosed with MS, service providers, family members, and friends must reinforce the expectation that people can stay on their jobs as long as they want to. By expecting success and orienting themselves toward functional abilities and capacities (rather than focusing on dysfunction, disability, and incapacitation), people with MS will be much more likely to retain and advance in their jobs.

Recommendation 9: Consult Assistive Technology Resources

Another promising factor in helping people with MS to retain and advance in their jobs is the use of appropriate assistive technology. As developmental advancements continue in this area, people with MS and other disabilities stand to be more independent, more productive in daily living and employment capacities, and less susceptible to the functional limitations associated with their conditions. Most states have federally sponsored technology assistance programs designed to help people with disabilities in identifying, acquiring, and learning to use assistive devices. Appendix D presents a state-by-state directory of those programs.

Recommendation 10: Conduct Research with Broad-Based National Samples

Employment interventions and other initiatives designed to increase the knowledge base concerning the career development implications of MS must be implemented at the national level. Far too many of the studies described in Chapters 2, 3, and 4 involved "micro-samples" that were restricted to circumscribed geographical areas. Multisite projects such as the Career Possibilities Project, the Job Raising Program, and Project Alliance need to be adopted on an ongoing, systematic basis.

In particular, a scientifically derived national sample of Americans with MS needs to be surveyed as to the incidence and prevalence of workplace discrimination facing people with MS in the ADA era. The field needs up-to-date information about (a) labor force participation, (b) the nature and type of workplace discrimination that people with MS experience, (c) how people with MS respond to perceived workplace discrimination, and (d) how effective Title I of the ADA is in remediating and resolving on-the-job discrimination for people with MS. Perhaps most importantly, a thorough investigation of respondents' self-reported employment discrimination experiences would enable researchers and service providers to develop interventions that are truly compatible with needs of the MS community.

Another content area where national-scale research is needed concerns the Social Security Administration's disability programs. We need to know how many people with MS nationwide receive Social Security Disability Insurance (SSDI) benefits, Supplemental Security Income (SSI), Medicare, and Medicaid. We also need to know how many people with MS couple Social Security benefits with short- and long-term disability insurance, workers' compensation benefits, and services and benefits from the United States Veterans Administration. Taken in aggregate, these disability-specific income maintenance and health insurance protections, which are predicated on the recipient being too disabled to work, keep millions of Americans with disabilities and thousands of people with MS out of the workforce. Worse yet, participation on Social Security disability roles constitutes a "life sentence" from a career development standpoint. According to Marini (26), less than 0.5 of 1.0 percent of Americans who receive SSDI benefits will ever resume substantial gainful employment.

Broad-based research with a geographically diverse national sample of Americans with MS is needed to answer the following questions related to Social Security:

1. How many Americans with MS receive SSDI and SSI benefits?
2. What is the cost to society in keeping these experienced, well-trained, and productive workers out of the labor force?
3. Have work incentives in the SSDI and SSI programs been helpful even on a small scale, in helping beneficiaries with MS reenter the work force?
4. What is the relationship between actual and perceived work disincentives in the SSI and SSDI programs and long-term employment outcomes?
5. What is the psychological and familial impact of the premature mass exodus from the labor force that accompanies the onset of MS?
6. What roles can physicians, nurses, social workers, psychologists, rehabilitation professionals, and employers play in dispelling the "too disabled to work" prophecy that keeps people with MS out of the workforce?
7. What career reentry interventions can be implemented to help people with MS who want to work in removing themselves from SSDI and SSI rolls?

Summary

Multiple sclerosis is an unpredictable disease that presents a wide range of adjustmental challenges for those who develop the illness. Typically occurring during the prime of life, MS disrupts and often impairs the person's ability to plan for the future, perform activities of daily living, work, and engage in virtually every other social role. Although the medical effects of MS are many, varied, and often severe, the capricious disease course and associated psychological impact make the illness a doubly difficult one to cope with, adjust to, and accept.

These factors combine to create a unique and imposing challenge for people with MS who wish to continue working. As a group, people with MS are well-educated, experienced, and productive employees, yet a high percentage of these individuals make a premature departure from the labor force.

Because existing service delivery mechanisms (e.g., vocational rehabilitation, independent living centers, workers' compensation) have had little success to date in addressing the complex career development needs of people with MS, researchers and service providers must join together to:

1. Further specify the seemingly unique impact that MS has on a person's employment prospects
2. Develop interventions to address those needs in a way that enables the person herself or himself to take primary responsibility for her ultimate employment success
3. Evaluate the effectiveness of those programs on a systematic, ongoing basis

The purpose of this book is to detail the medical, demographical, psychological, and social factors that affect the employment status of people with MS. It also sought to describe model assessment and intervention strategies that have demonstrated the potential to assist people with MS in seeking, securing, and maintaining employment. Coupling that information with knowledge of the ADA, the Family and Medical Leave Act, the Health Insurance Portability and Accountability Act, the Consolidated Omnibus Budget Reconciliation Act, and the Social Security Act will afford people with MS the best opportunity to establish and continue in their careers, thereby enabling them to enjoy the well-documented economic, personal, and social benefits of active participation in the world of work.

References

1. Mullins, J.A., Jr., Rumrill, P.D., Jr., & Roessler, R.T. (1996). The role of the rehabilitation placement consultant in the ADA era. *Work: A Journal of Prevention, Assessment, and Rehabilitation* 6(1), 3–10.
2. LaRocca, N. (1995). *Employment and multiple sclerosis.* New York: National Multiple Sclerosis Society.
3. Rumrill, P. (2006). Help to stay at work: Vocational rehabilitation strategies for people with multiple sclerosis. *Multiple Sclerosis in Focus, 7,* 14–18.
4. Fraser, R., Kraft, G., Ehde, D., & Johnson, K. (2006). *The multiple sclerosis workbook: Living fully with MS.* Oakland, CA. New Harbinger Publications.
5. Roessler, R., Rumrill, P., & Hennessey, M. (2002). *Employment concerns of people with multiple sclerosis: Building a national employment agenda.* New York: National Multiple Sclerosis Society.
6. Sumner, G. (1995). *Project Alliance: A job retention program for employees with chronic illnesses and their employers.* Unpublished manuscript.
7. Roessler, R., & Rumrill, P. (2003). Multiple sclerosis and employment barriers: A systemic perspective on diagnosis and intervention. *Work: A Journal of Prevention, Assessment and Rehabilitation 21*(1), 17–23.
8. DuPont Corporation (1990). *Equal to the task II; DuPont survey of employment of people with disabilities.* Wilmington, DE: E.I. DuPont de Nemours.

9. Federation Employment and Guidance Services (1957). *Survey of employers' practices and policies in the hiring of physically impaired workers* (HEW Vocational Rehabilitation Grant). New York: Federation Employment and Guidance Services.

10. Schletzer, V.M., Dawis, R.V., England, G.W., & Lofquist, L. (1961). *Attitudinal barriers to employment* (OVR Special Report RD—422). Minneapolis: University of Minnesota Industrial Relations Center.

11. Shapiro, J.P. (1993). No pity: *People with disabilities forging a new civil rights movement.* New York: Random House.

12. Zunker, V.G. (1994). *Foundations of career counseling: Applied concepts of life planning.* Pacific Grove, CA: Brooks/Cole Publishing.

13. Hennessey, M., & Rumrill, P. (2001).Overview of multiple sclerosis. In P. Rumrill & M. Hennessey (Eds.), *Multiple sclerosis: A guide for health care and rehabilitation professionals.* Springfield, IL: Charles C Thomas, pp. 3–22.

14. Ketelaer, P., Crijns, H., Gausin, J., & Bouwen, R. (1993). *Multiple sclerosis and employment: Synthesis report.* Brussels: Belgian Ministry of Labour and Employment.

15. Bellini, J., & Rumrill, P. (1999). Perspectives on scientific inquiry: Validity in rehabilitation research. *Journal of Vocational Rehabilitation, 13*(2), 131–138.

16. Bellini, J. (2001). Implementation and evaluation of the order of selection mandate in state vocational rehabilitation agencies. In P. Rumrill, J. Bellini, & L.Koch (Eds.), *Emerging issues in rehabilitation counseling: Perspectives on the new millennium.* Springfield, IL: Charles C Thomas Publisher, pp.122–146.

17. Roessler, R.T., & Bolton, B. (1985). Employment patterns of former vocational rehabilitation clients and implications for rehabilitation practice. *Rehabilitation Counseling Bulletin, 28*(3), 179–187.

18. Neubert, D.A., Tilson, G.P., & Ianacone, R.N. (1989). Postsecondary transition needs and employment patterns of individuals with mild disabilities. *Exceptional Children, 55*(6), 494–500.

19. Gibbs, W.E. (1990) Alternative measures to evaluate the impact of vocational rehabilitation services. *Rehabilitation Counseling Bulletin, 34*(1), 33–43.

20. United States General Accounting Office (1993). Vocational rehabilitation: *Evidence for federal program's effectiveness mixed.* Washington, DC: United States Accounting Office.

21. Equal Employment Opportunity Commission and Department of Justice (1991). *The Americans with Disabilities Act handbook.* Washington, DC: United States Government Printing Office.

22. Schriner, K.F., Rumrill, P.D., & Parlin, R. (1995). Rethinking disability policy: Equity in the ADA era and the meaning of specialized services for people with disabilities. *Journal of the Health and Human Services Administration, 17*(4), 478–500.

23. Rubin, S., & Roessler, R. (2001). *Foundations of the vocational rehabilitation process.* Austin: PRO-ED.

24. Wehmen, P. (2006). *Life beyond the classroom.* Baltimore: Paul H. Brooks Publishing.

25. Rumrill, P.D., Jr., & Gordon, S.E. (1994). Integrated career development services for college students with disabilities: From philosophy to practice. In D. Ryan & M. McCarthy (Eds.), *NASPA monograph: Disability issues in higher education.* Washington, DC: National Association of Student Personnel Administrators, pp. 111–124.

26. Marini, I. (2003). What rehabilitation counselors should know to assist Social Security beneficiaries in becoming employed. *Work, 21*(1), 37–44.

Vocational Rehabilitation Agencies

Alabama
Department of Rehabilitation Services
P.O. Box 11586
Montgomery, AL 36111-0586
Phone: 334-281-8780
Toll-free: 800-441-7607
Toll-free restrictions: Alabama residents only
FAX: 334-281-1973
TTY: 888-737-2032
E-mail: ssivers@rehab.state.al.us
Website: www.rehab.stat.al.us/

Alaska
Division of Vocational Rehabilitation
Department of Labor and Workforce Development
Suite A
801 West 10th Street
Juneau, AK 99801-1849
Phone: 907-465-2814
Toll-free: 800-478-2815
Toll-free restrictions: Alaska residents only

FAX: 907-465-2856
TTY: 907-465-2814
E-mail: mark_dale@labor.state.ak.us
Website: www.labor.state.ak.us/dvr/home/htm

Arizona
Rehabilitation Services Administration
Department of Economic Security
2nd Floor, Site Code 930A
1739 West Jefferson, NW
Phoenix, AZ 85007-3202
Phone: 602-542-3332
Toll-free: 800-563-1221
FAX: 602-542-3778
TTY: 602-542-6049
E-mail: klenadowsky@azdes.gov or arsa@azdes.gov
Website: www.de.state.az.us/rsa

Arkansas
Arkansas Rehabilitation Services
1616 Brookwood Drive
P.O. Box 3781
Little Rock, AR 72203-3781
Phone: 501-296-1616
Toll-free: 800-330-0632
FAX: 501-296-1655
TTY: 501-296-1669
E-mail: kmusteen@ars.state.ar.us or rptrevino@ars.state.ar.us
Website: www.arsinfo.org/

Division of Services for the Blind
State Department of Human Services
P.O. Box 3237
Little Rock AR 72203-3237
Phone: 501-682-5463
Toll-free: 800-960-9270
Toll restriction: Arkansas residents only
FAX: 501-682-0366
TTY: 501-682-0093

E-mail: Dorothy.brooks@arkansas.gov or jim.hudson@arkansas.gov
Website: www.state.ar.us/dhhs/dsb/NEWDSB/index.htm

California
Department of Rehabilitation
2000 Evergreen Street
Sacramento, CA 95815
Phone: 916-263-8987
FAX: 916-263-7474
TTY: 916-263-7477
E-mail: publicaffairs@dor.ca.gov
Website: www.dor.ca.gov

Colorado
Division of Vocational Rehabilitation
State Department of Human Services
4th Floor
1575 Sherman Street
Denver, CO 80203
Phone: 303-866-4150
FAX: 303-866-4905
TTY: 303-866-4150
E-mail: nancy.smith@state.co.us
Website: www.cdhs.state.co.us/index.htm

Connecticut
Bureau of Rehabilitation Services
State Department of Social Services
11th Floor
25 Sigourney Street
Hartford, CT 06106-2055
Phone: 860-424-4844
Toll-free: 800-537-2549
Toll-free restrictions: Connecticut residents only
FAX: 860-424-4850
TTY: 800-424-4839
E-mail: evelyn.knight@po.state.ct.us
Website: www.brs.state.ct.us/

Vocational Rehabilitation Division
State Board of Education and Services for the Blind
184 Windsor Avenue
Windsor, CT 06095
Phone: 860-602-4008
Toll-free: 800-842-4510
Toll-free restrictions: Connecticut residents only
FAX: 860-602-4030
TTY: 860-602-4221
E-mail: brian.sigman@po.state.ct.us or BESB@PO.STATE.CT.US
Website: www.ct.gov/besb/site/default.asp

Delaware

Division of Vocational Rehabilitation
State Department of Labor
4425 North Street
P.O. Box 9969
Wilmington, DE 19809-0969
Phone: 302-761-8275
FAX: 302-761-6611
TTY: 302-761-8275
E-mail: edwom/tps@state.de.us or andrea.guest@state.de.us

Vocational and Rehabilitation Agency
Division for the Visually Impaired
DHSS Campus, Biggs Building
1901 North DuPont Highway
New Castle, DE 19702-1199
Phone: 302-255-9800
FAX: 302-255-9964
E-mail: bob.goodhart@state.de.us or Cynthia.lovell@state.de.us
Website: www.delawareworks.com/dvr/welcome.shtml

District of Columbia

Rehabilitation Services Administration
Department of Human Services
10th Floor
810 First Street
Washington, DC 20002

Phone: 202-442-8663
FAX: 202-442-8742
E-mail: elizabeth.parker@dc.gov

Florida
Division of Vocational Rehabilitation
Florida Department of Education
Building A
2002 Old St. Augustine Road
Tallahassee, FL 32301-4862
Phone: 850-245-3399
Toll-free: 800-451-4327
Toll-free restrictions: Florida residents only
FAX: 850-245-3316
TTY: 850-245-3399
E-mail: Bill.Palmer@vr.fldoe.prg or Sue.Yates@vr.fldoe.org
Website: www.rehabworks.org

Vocational Rehabilitation Agency
Division of Blind Services
Turlington Building
325 West Gaines Street
Tallahassee, FL 32399-2050
Phone: 850-245-0300
Toll-free: 800-342-1828
Toll-free restrictions: Florida residents only
FAX: 850-245-0360
E-mail: Stephanie.wilson@dbs.fldoe.org of craig.kiser@dbs.fldoe.org
Website: www.state.fl.us/dbs/index.shtml

Georgia
Rehabilitation Services
State Department of Labor
Suite 510
418 Andrew Young International Boulevard, NE
Atlanta, GA 30303-1751
Phone: 404-232-3910
FAX: 404-232-3910
TTY: 404-232-3911

E-mail: rehab@dol.state.ga.us or pegge.rosser@dol.state.ga.us
Website: www.vocrehabga.org

Hawaii

Vocational and Rehabilitation Agency
Vocational Rehabilitation Services for the Blind Division
Kapolei State Office Building, Room 515
Kapolei, HI 96707
Phone: 808-692-7719
FAX: 808-692-7727
TTY: 808-692-7715
E-mail: jnoland@dhs.hawaii.gov or jcordova@dhs.hawaii.gov
Website: www.hawaii.gov/dhs/self-sufficiency/vr/

Idaho

Division of Vocational Rehabilitation
Len B. Jordan Building
Room 150
Boise, ID 83720-0096
Phone: 208-334-3390
FAX: 208-334-5305
E-mail: rthomea@vr.idaho.gov or mgraham@vr.idaho.gov
Website: www.vr.idaho.gov/

Vocational Rehabilitation Agency
Idaho Commission for the Blind and Visually Impaired
341 West Washington Street
Boise, ID 83702-0012
Phone: 208-334-3220
Toll-free: 800-542-8688
Toll-free restrictions: Idaho residents only
FAX: 208-334-2963
E-mail: aroan@icbvi.idaho.gov
Website: www.icbvi.state.id.us/

Illinois

Division of Rehabilitation Services
State Department of Human Services
2nd Floor
100 South Grand Avenue

Springfield, IL 62762
Phone: 217-557-7048
Toll-free: 800-843-6154
Toll-free restrictions: Illinois residents only
FAX: 217-558-4270
TTY: 888-440-8990
E-mail: Robert.kilbury@illinois.gov
Website: www.illinois.gov

Indiana

Bureau of Rehabilitation Services
Division of Disability and Rehabilitative Services
402 West Washington Street
P.O. Box 7083
Indianapolis, IN 46207-7083
Phone: 317-234-4475
Toll-free: 800-545-7763
Toll-free restrictions: Indiana residents only
FAX: 317-232-6478
TTY: 8317-232-1427
E-mail: Michael.Hedden@fssa.in.gov
Website: www.in.gov/fssa/disability/services/vr/index.html

Iowa

Vocational Rehabilitation Agency
Iowa Department for the Blind
524 Fourth Street
Des Moines, IA 50309-2264
Phone: 515-281-1334
Toll-free: 800-362-2587
Toll-free restrictions: Iowa residents only
FAX: 515-281-1263
TTY: 515-281-1355
E-mail: harris.allen@blind.state.ia.us
Website: www.blind.state.ia.us/

Vocational Rehabilitation Services
State Department of Education
510 East 12th Street

Dees Moines, IA 50139-0240
Phone: 515-281-4211
Toll-free: 800-532-1486
FAX: 515-281-4703
TTY: 515-281-4211
E-mail: www.mccord@iowa.gov or Stephen.wooderson@iowa.gov
Website: www.ivrs.iowa.gov/

Kansas

Rehabilitation Services
Department of Social and Rehabilitation Services
Suite 150
3640 South West Topeka Boulevard
Topeka, KS 66611-2376
Phone: 785-267-5301
Toll-free: 888-369-4777
Toll-free restrictions: Kansas residents only
FAX: 785-267-0263
TTY: 785-267-0352
E-mail: rehab.mail@srs.ks.gov
Website: www.srskansas.org/rehab/

Kentucky

Kentucky Office of Vocational Rehabilitation
209 Saint Clair Street
Frankfort, KY 40601
Phone: 502-564-4440
Toll-free: 800-372-7172
Toll-free restrictions: KY residents only
FAX: 502-564-6745
TTY: 502-564-6817
E-mail: ralphm.clark@ky.gov
Website: www.ovr.ky.gov/index.htm

Vocational an Rehabilitation Agency
State Office for the Blind
209 Saint Clair Street
P.O. Box 757
Frankfort, KY 40601

Phone: 502-564-4754
Toll-free: 800-321-6668
FAX: 502-564-2951
TTY: 502-564-2929
E-mail: marciam.egbert@ky.gov or Stephen.johnson@ky.gov
Website: www.blind.ky.gov

Louisiana
Rehabilitation Services
State Department of Social Services
8225 Florida Blvd.
Baton Rouge, LA 70806-4834
Phone: 225-925-4131
Toll-free: 800-737-2958
Toll-free restrictions: LA residents only
FAX: 225-925-4184
TTY: 225-925-4131
E-mail: chymel@dss.state.la.us or jwallace@dss.state.la.us
Website: www.dss.state.la.us/departments/lrs/index.html

Maine
Division of Vocational Rehabilitation
Maine Department of Labor
Bureau of Rehabilitation Services
150 State House Station
Augusta, ME 04333-0150
Phone: 207-624-5950
Toll-free: 800-698-4440
Toll-free restrictions: ME residents only
FAX: 207-624-5980
TTY: 207-624-5965
E-mail: penny.plourde@maine.gov
Website: www.state.me.us/rehab/

Vocational and Rehabilitation Agency
Division for the Blind and Visually Impaired
State Department of Labor
150 State House Station
Augusta, ME 04333-0150

Phone: 207-623-7956
Toll-free: 800-698-4440
Toll-free restrictions: ME residents only
FAX: 207-624-5980
TTY: 888-755-0023
E-mail: paul.e.cot@maine.gov or Harold.j.lewis@maine.gov
Website: www.state.me.us/rehab/

Maryland

Division of Rehabilitation Services
State Department of Education
2301 Argonne Drive
Baltimore, MD 21218-1696
Phone: 410-554-9385
Toll-free: 888-554-0334
FAX: 410-554-9412
TTY: 410-554-9411
E-mail: dneff@dors.state.me.us or rburns@dors.state.md.us
Website: www.dors.state.md.us

Massachusetts

Rehabilitation Commission
Fort Pointe Place
27 Wormwood Street
Boston, MA 02210-1606
Phone: 617-204-3600
Toll-free: 800-245-6543
Toll restrictions: MA residents only
FAX: 617-727-1354
TTY: 800-245-6543
E-mail: kasper.goshgarian@mrc.state.ma.us or elmer.bartels@mrc.state.
    ma.us
Website: www.state.ma.is.mrc

Vocational Rehabilitation Agency
Massachusetts Commission for the Blind
48 Boylston Street
Boston, MA 02216-4718
Phone: 617-727-5550 x7503

Toll-free: 800-392-6450
Toll-free restrictions: MA residents only
FAX: 617-626-7685
TTY: 800-392-6556
E-mail: susan.lavin@state.ma.us or david.govostes@state.ma.us
Website: www.state.ma.us/mcb

Michigan

Department of Human Services
Disability Determination Services
P.O. Box 30011
Lansing, MI 48909
Phone: 517-241-7799
Toll-free: 800-366-3404
Toll-free restrictions: MI residents only
FAX: 517-335-7771
E-mail: Kelly.tullar@ssa.gov or byron.haskins@ssa.gov
Website: www.michigan.gov/dhs

Michigan Commission for the Blind
201 North Washington Square
P.O. Box 30652
Lansing, MI 48909-2062
Phone: 517-373-2062
Toll-free: 800-292-4200
Toll-free restrictions: MI residents only
FAX: 517-335-5140
TTY: 888-864-1212
E-mail: cannonp@michigan.gov

Rehabilitation Services
Department of Labor and Economic Growth
201 North Washington Square
P.O. Box 30010
Lansing, MI 48909
Phone: 517-373-3390
Toll-free: 800-605-6722
Toll-free restrictions: MI residents only
FAX: 517-335-7277

TTY: 888-605-6722
E-mail: shamsiddeenj@michigan.gov
Website: www.michigan.gov/mdcd/0,1607,7-122-25392---,00.html

Minnesota

Department of Employment and Economic Development
State Services for the Blind
Suite 240
2200 University Avenue West
Saint Paul, MN 55114-1840
Phone: 651-642-0500
Toll-free: 800-652-9000
Toll-free restrictions: MN residents only
FAX: 651-649-5927
TTY: 651-642-0506
E-mail: chuk.hamilton@state.mn.us
Website: www.mnssb.org/

Rehabilitation Services
State Department of Employment and Economic Development
First National Bank Building
332 Minnesota Street, Suite E200
Saint Paul, MN 55101-1351
Phone: 651-296-7510
Toll-free: 800-328-9095
Toll-free restrictions: MN residents only
FAX: 651-297-5159
TTY: 651-296-3900
E-mail: kim.peck@state.mn.us or paul.moe@state.mn.us
Website: www.deed.state.mn.us/rehab/rehab.htm

Mississippi

Department of Rehabilitation Services
Office of Vocational Rehabilitation for the Blind
P.O. Box 1698
Jackson, MS 39215-1698
Phone: 601-853-5100
Toll-free: 800-443-1000

FAX: 601-853-5158
TTY: 601-853-5310
E-mail: Michael.gandy@mdrs.state.ms.us or bmcmillan@mdrs.state.ms.us
Website: www.mdrs.state.ms.us/

Missouri

Division of Vocational Rehabilitation
State Department of Elementary and Secondary Education
3024 Dupont Circle
Jefferson City, MO 65109-2320
Phone: 573-751-3251
Toll-free: 877-222-8963
FAX: 573-751-1441
TTY: 573-751-0881
E-mail: patsy.helmig@vr.dese.mo.gov or jeanne.loyd@vr.dese.mo.gov
Website: www.vr.dese.mo.gov

Rehabilitation Services for the Blind
Family Support Division
615 Howerton Court
P.O. Box 2320
Jefferson City, MO 65102-2320
Phone: 573-751-4249
FAX: 573-751-4984
TTY: 573-592-6004
E-mail: Michael.c.fester@dss.mo.gov

Montana

Department of Public Health and Human Services
Disability Services Division
111 North Sanders, Room 307
P.O. Box 4210
Helena, MT 59604-4210
Phone: 406-444-2590
Toll-free: 877-296-1197
FAX: 406-444-3632
TTY: 406-444-2590
E-mail: dphhstech@mt.gov. or jmathews@mt.gov
Website: www.dphhs.mt.gov/dsd

Nebraska

Commission for the Blind and Visually Impaired
Suite 100
4600 Valley Road
Lincoln, NE 68510-4844
Phone: 402-471-2891
Toll-free: 877-809-2419
Toll-free restrictions: NE residents only
FAX: 402-471-3009
E-mail: val.perry@ncbvi.ne.gov or pearl.vanzandt@ncbvi.ne.gov
Website: www.ncbvi.ne.gov

Division of Vocational Rehabilitation Services
State Department of Education
301 Centennial Mall South, 6th Floor
P.O. Box 94987
Lincoln, NE 68509-4987
Phone: 402-471-3644
Toll-free: 877-637-3422
Toll-free restrictions: NE residents only
FAX: 402-471-0788
TTY: 402-471-3644
E-mail: vr_stateoffice@vocrehab.state.ne.us or frank.lloyd@vr.ne.gov
Website: www.vocrehab.state.ne.us/

Nevada

Department of Employment, Training, and Rehabilitation
Rehabilitation Division
1370 South Curry Street
Carson City, NV 89703-5146
Phone: 775-684-4040
FAX: 775-684-4184
TTY: 775-684-8400
E-mail: detrvr@nvdetr.org or cablackmore@nvdetr.org
Website: detr.state.nv.us/rehab/reh_index.htm

New Hampshire

Division of Adult Learning and Rehabilitation
Vocational Rehabilitation

188

State Department of Education
21 South Fruit Street, Suite 20
Concord, NH 03301-2428
Phone: 603-271-3471
Toll-free: 800-299-1647
Toll-free restrictions: NH residents only
FAX: 603-271-7095
TTY: 603-271-3471
E-mail: shadley@ed.state.nh.us or pleather@ed.state.nh.us
Website: www.ed.state.nh.us/Education/doe/organization/
   adultlearning/VR

New Jersey

Commission for the Blind and the Visually Impaired
State Department of Human Services
153 Halsey Street, 6th Floor
P.O. Box 47017
Newark, NJ 07101
Phone: 973-648-3333
FAX: 973-648-7364
TTY: 973-648-4559
E-mail: greg.patty@dhs.state.nj.us or vito.desantis@dhs.state.nj.us
Website: www.state.nj.us/humanservices/cbvi/dhscov.htm

Division of Vocational Rehabilitation Services
Department of Labor and Workforce Development
P.O. Box 398
Trenton, NJ 08625-0398
Phone: 609-292-5987
Toll-free: 866-871-7867
FAX: 609-292-4033
TTY: 609-292-2919
E-mail: Thomas.jennings@dol.state.nj.us
Website: www.state.nj.us/labor.dvrs/vrsindex.html

New Mexico

Division of Vocational Rehabilitation
State Department of Education
Building D

435 Saint Michaels Drive
Santa Fe, NM 87505
Phone: 505-954-8500
Toll-free: 800-224-7005
FAX: 505-954-8562
TTY: 505-292-0454 (Relay New Mexico)
E-mail: Richard.smith@state.nm.us or doris.chavez@state.nm.us
Website: www.dvrgetsjobs.com/

New Mexico Commission for the Blind
Building 4, Suite 100
2905 Rodeo Park Drive, East
Santa Fe, NM87505
Phone: 505-476-4479
Toll-free: 888-513-7968
Toll-free restrictions: NM residents only
FAX: 505-476-4475
TTY: 505-476-6407
E-mail: Evelyn.Blair@state.nm.us or Greg.Trapp@state.nm.us
Website: www.cfb.state.nm.us/

New York
Special Education and Vocational Rehabilitation Agency
State Department of Education
Vocational and Educational Services for Individuals with Disabilities
One Commerce Plaza, Room 1606
Albany, NY 12234-2822
Phone: 518-474-2714
FAX: 518-474-8802
TTY: 518-474-5652
E-mail: rcort@mail.nysed.gov
Website: www.vesid.nysed.gov/

State Commission or the Blind and Visually Handicapped
Office of Children and Family Services
South Building, Room 201
52 Washington Street
Renssealaer, NY 12144-2796
Phone: 518-474-7299

FAX: 518-486-5819
TTY: 518-474-7501
E-mail: brian.daniels@dfa.state.ny.us

North Carolina

Division of Services for the Blind
Department of Health and Human Services
2601 Mail Services Center
Raleigh, NC 27699-2601
Phone: 919-733-9822
Toll-free: 866-222-1546
FAX: 919-733-9769
TTY: 919-733-9700
E-mail: Debbie.Jackson@ncmail.net
Website: www.ncdhhs.gov/dsb

Division of Vocational and Rehabilitation Services
Department of Health and Human Services
2801 Mail Services Center
Raleigh, NC 27699-2601
Phone: 919-855-3500
FAX: 919-733-7968
TTY: 919-855-3579
E-mail: dvr.info@ncmail.net or Linda.Harrington@ncmail.net
Website: dvr.dhhs.state.nc.us/

North Dakota

North Dakota Department of Human Services
Disability Services Division
Prairie Hill Plaza
1237 West Divided Avenue, Suite 1B
Bismarck, ND 58501-1208
Phone: 7001-328-8950
Toll-free: 800-755-2745
FAX: 7001-328-8969
TTY: 701-328-8968
E-mail: dgsds@nd.gov or wbye@nd.gov
Website: www.nd.gov/humanservices/services/disabilities/

Ohio

Rehabilitation Services Commission
400 East Campus View Blvd
Columbus, OH 43235-4606
Phone: 614-438-1210
Toll-free: 800-282-4536 x1210
Toll-free restrictions: Ohio residents only
FAX: 614-785-5010
TTY: 614-785-5048
E-mail: beverly.jennings@rsc.state.oh.us or
   John.Connelly@rsc.state.oh.us
Website: www.rsc.ohio.gov/

Oklahoma

State Department of Rehabilitation Services
Suite 500
3535 NW 58th Street
Oklahoma City, OK 73112
Phone: 405-951-3400
Toll-free: 800-282-4536 x1210
Toll-free restriction: OK residents only
FAX: 405-951-3529
TTY: 405-951-3400
E-mail: jharlan@drs.state.ok.us or lparker@drs.state.ok.us
Website: www.okrehab.org/

Oregon

Office of Vocational Rehabilitation Services
State Department of Human Services
Children, Adult, and Family Services
500 Summer Street NE, E-87
Salem, OR 97301-1120
Phone: 503-945-5880
Toll-free: 877-277-0513
FAX: 503-947-5025
TTY: 503-945-5894
E-mail: stephaine.taylor@state.or.us or vrinfo@state.or.us
Website: egov.oregon.gov/DHS/vr/index.shtml

Oregon Commission for the Blind
535 SE 12th Street
Portland, OR 97214
Phone: 971-673-1588
Toll-free: 888-202-5463
Toll-free restrictions: OR residents only
FAX: 971-673-1570
E-mail: ocb@state.or.us or Linda.mock@state.or.us
Website: www.cfb.state.or.us

Pennsylvania

Office of Vocational Rehabilitation
Department of Labor and Industry
1521 North Sixth Street
Harrisburg, PA 17102
Phone: 717-787-5244
Toll-free: 800-442-6351
Toll-free restrictions: PA residents only
FAX: 717-783-5221
TTY: 717-787-4885
E-mail: dli@state.ppa.us or wgannon@state.pa.us
Website: www.dli.state.pa.us/landi/cwp/view.asp?a=128&q=61197

Vocational and Rehabilitation Agency
Bureau of Blindness and Visual Services
Department of Labor and Industry
1521 North Sixth Street
Harrisburg, PA 17102
Phone: 717-787-6176
Toll-free: 800-622-2842
Toll-free restrictions: PA residents only
FAX: 717-772-1629
TTY: 717-787-4885
E-mail: lushumaker@state.pa.us
Website: www.dli.state.pa.us/landi/cwp/view.asp?

Rhode Island

Office of Rehabilitation Services
Department of Human Services

40 Fountain Street
Providence, RI 02903
Phone: 401-421-7005
FAX: 401-222-3574
TTY: 401-421-7016
E-mail: rcarroll@ors.ri.gov
Website: www.ors.ri.gov/

South Carolina

Commission for the Blind
1430 Confederate Avenue
P.O. Box 2467
Columbia, SC 29202-0079
Phone: 803-898-8700
Toll-free: 800-922-2222
Toll-free restrictions: SC residents only
FAX: 803-898-8852
E-mail: Ljohnston@sccb.sc.gov or publicinfo@sccb.sc.gov
Website: sccb.state.sc.us

Vocational Rehabilitation Department
1410 Boston Avenue
P.O. Box 15
West Columbia, SC 29171-0015
Phone: 803-896-6504
Toll-free: 800-832-7526
Toll-free restrictions: SC residents only
FAX: 803-896-6529
TTY: 803-896-6666
E-mail: info@scvrd.state.sc.us or lcbryant@scvrd.state.sc.us
Website: www.scvrd.net

South Dakota

Division of Rehabilitation Services
Department of Human Services
500 East Capital
East Highway 34
Pierre, SD 57501-5070
Phone: 605-773-3195

Toll-free: 800-265-9684
FAX: 605-773-5483
TTY: 605-773-5990
E-mail: becky.blume@state.sd.us or grady.kickul@state.sd.us
Website: dhs.sd.gov/drs/

Division of Services to the Blind and Visually Impaired
Hillsview Plaza
c/o 500 East Capital
3800 East Highway
Pierre, SD 57501-5070
Phone: 605-773-4644
Toll-free: 800-265-9684
Toll-free restrictions: South Dakota residents only
FAX: 605-773-5483
TTY: 605-773-4644
E-mail: eric.weiss@state.sd.usorgaye.mattke@state.sd.us
Website: dhs.sd.gov/sbvi/

Tennessee
Vocational Rehabilitation Services
Department of Human Services
Citizens Plaza State Office Building, 15th Floor
400 Deaderick Street
Nashville, TN 37248-0060
Phone: 615-313-4714
FAX: 615-741-4165
TTY: 6115-313-5695
E-mail: Andrea.Cooper@state.tn.us
Website: tennessee.gov/humanserv/rehab/vrs.htm

Texas
Department of Assistive and Rehabilitative Services
Division of Rehabilitation Services
Suite 310
4800 North Lamar Blvd
Austin, TX 78756-3178
Phone: 512-377-0602
Toll-free: 800-628-5115

Toll-free restrictions: TX residents only
FAX: 512-377-0682
TTY: 512-377-0573
E-mail: dars.inquires@dars.state.tx.us or
  Barbara.j.madrigal@dars.state.tx.us
Website: www.dars.state.tx.us

Department of Assistive and Rehabilitative Services
Division of Rehabilitation Services
Suite 5667
4900 North Lamar Blvd
Austin, TX 78751-2399
Phone: 512-424-4220
Toll-free: 800-628-5115
FAX: 512-424-4277
TTY: 800-628-5115
E-mail: dars.inquires@dars.state.tx.us
Website: www.dars.state.tx.us/

Utah

State Office of Rehabilitation
250 East 500 South
P.O. Box 144200
Salt Lake City, UT 84114-4200
Phone: 801-538-7530
Toll-free: 800-473-7530
Toll-free restrictions: UT residents only
FAX: 801-538-7522
TTY: 801-538-7530
E-mail: duchida@utah.gov or rthelin@utah.gov
Website: www.usor.utah.gov/

Vocational and Rehabilitation Agency
Division of Services for the Blind and Visually Impaired
State Office of Rehabilitation
250 North 1950 West, Suite B
Salt Lake City, UT 84116-7902
Phone: 801-323-4343
Toll-free: 800-284-1823

196

Toll-free restrictions: UT residents only
FAX: 801-323-4396
TTY: 801-323-4395
E-mail: mberry@utah.gov
Website: www.usor.utah.gov/dsbvi.htm

Vermont

Division of the Blind and Visually Impaired
Agency of Human Services
Weeks IC, Room 109
103 South Main Street
Waterbury, VT 05671-2304
Phone: 802-241-2210
Toll-free: 888-405-5005
Toll-free restrictions: VT residents only
FAX: 802-241-2128
E-mail: loreen.guyette@dail.state.vt.us or fred.jones@dail.state.vt.us
Website: www.dad.state.vt.us/dbvi/

Vocational Rehabilitation Division
Agency of Human Services
Weeks Building, 1A
103 South Main Street
Waterbury, VT 05671-2303
Phone: 802-241-2186
Toll-free: 866-879-6757
Toll-free restrictions: VT residents only
FAX: 802-241-3359
TTY: 802-241-1455
E-mail: diane.dalmasse@dail.state.vt.us
Website: vocrehab.vermont.gov/

Virginia

Department for the Blind and Vision Impaired
397 Azalea Avenue
Richmond, VA 23227-3623
Phone: 804-371-3140
Toll-free: 800-622-2155
Toll-free restrictions: VA residents only

FAX: 804-371-3351
TTY: 804-371-3140
E-mail: susan.payne@dbvi.virginia.gov or William.pega@dbvi.virginia.gov
Website: www.vdbvi.org

Department of Rehabilitation Services
8004 Franklin Farms Drive
Richmond, VA 23229
Phone: 804-662-7000
Toll-free: 800-552-5019
Toll-free restrictions: VA residents only
FAX: 804-662-7644
TTY: 804-662-9040
E-mail: drs@drs.state.va.us or Jim.rothrock@drs.virginia.gov
Website: www.vadrs.org/

Washington

Department of Services for the Blind
P.O. Box 40933
Olympia, WA 98504-0933
Phone: 209-721-6400
Toll-free: 800-552-7103
Toll-free restrictions: WA residents only
FAX: 206-721-4103
TTY: 206-721-4056
E-mail: information@dsb.wa.gov or loudurand@dsb.wa.gov
Website: www.dsb.wa.gov/

Division of Vocational Rehabilitation
Department of Social and Health Services
P.O. Box 45340
Olympia, WA 98504-5340
Phone: 360-725-3610
Toll-free: 800-637-5627
Toll-free restrictions: WA residents only
FAX: 360-438-8011
E-mail: ruttllm@dshs.wa.gov
Website: www1.dshs.wa.gov/dvr/

West Virginia

Division of Rehabilitation Services
P.O. Box 50890
State Capitol
Charleston, WV 25305-0890
Phone: 304-766-4601
Toll-free: 800-642-8207
FAX: 304-766-4905
TTY: 304-766-4965
E-mail: donna@mail.drs.state.wv.us or Debbiel@wvdrs.org

Wisconsin

Division of Vocational Rehabilitation
Department of Workforce Development
201 East Washington Avenue, Suite A100
P.O. Box 7852
Madison, WI 53707-7852
Phone: 608-261-0050
Toll-free: 800-442-3477
Toll-free restrictions: WI residents only
FAX: 608-266-1133
TTY: 888-877-5939
E-mail: dwddvr@dwd.state.wi.is or
    charlene.dwyer@dwd.state.wi.us
Website: dwd.wisconsin.gov/dvr/

Wyoming

Division of Vocational Rehabilitation
Department of Workforce Services
Herschler Building
122 West 25th Street
Cheyenne, WY 82002
Phone: 307-777-7389
FAX: 307-777-5939
TTY: 307-777-7386
E-mail: jmcint@state.wy.us
Website: www.wyomingworkforce.org

Vocational Rehabilitation Agencies in the US Territories

American Samoa
Division of Vocational Rehabilitation
Department of Human Social Services
P.O. Box 501521
Pago Pago, AS 96799-4561
Phone: 684-699-1371
FAX: 684-699-1376
E-mail: apisap26@yahoo.com

Commonwealth of the Northern Mariana Islands
CNMI Office of Vocational Rehabilitation
Office of the Governor
P.O. Box 501521
Navy Hill, Building #N2
Saipan, MP 96950
Phone: 670-322-6537/8
FAX: 670-322-6563
TTY: 670-322-6449
E-mail: voc.rehab@saipan.com or ovr@ovr.gov.mp
Website: www.ovr.gov.mp/about.asp

Guam
Division of Vocational Rehabilitation
1313 Central Avenue
Tiyan, GU 96913
Phone: 671-475-4200
FAX: 671-475-4661
TTY: 671-477-8642
E-mail: dvrsana@ite.net or webteam@mail.gov.gu
website: bit.guam.gov/Home/tabid/747/Default.aspx

Puerto Rico
Vocational Rehabilitation Administration
Department of Labor and Human Services
P.O. Box 191118
San Juana, PR 00919-1118

Phone: 787-727-0445
FAX: 787-728-8070
TTY: 787-268-3735
E-mail: dorcas@vra.gobierno.pr
Website: www.dtrh.gobierno.pr/

Virgin Islands
Division of Disabilities and Rehabilitation Services
Knud Hansen Complex, Building A
1303 Hospital Ground
St. Thomas, VI 00802
Phone: 340-774-0930 x4190
FAX: 340-774-7773
TTY: 340-776-2043
E-mail: plaskettb@islands.vi or bcplaskett@hotmail.com

Disability and Business Technical Assistance Centers (DBTACs)

VCU DBTAC Coordination, Outreach, and Research Center
1112 East Clay Street
P.O. Box 980330
Richmond, VA 23298-0330
Phone: 804-827-0917
Fax: 804-828-1321
Website: www.dbtac.vcu.edu/ar/educators
For ADA technical assistance, contact your local center
  at 800-949-4232

Region 1 (CT, ME, MA, NH, RI, VT)
DBTAC—New England ADA Center
Adaptive Environments Center, Inc.
180-200 Portland Street
1st Floor
Boston, MA 02114
Phone (V/TTY): 617-695-1225
Fax: 617-482-8099
E-mail: adainfo@newenglandada.org
Website: www.adaptiveenvironments.org/neada/site/home

Region 2 (NJ, NY, PR, VI)

DBTAC—Northeast ADA Center
Cornell University
DBTAC—Northeast ADA Center
331 Ives
Ithaca, NY 14853-3901
Phone: 607-255-8348
TTY: 607-255-6686
Fax: 607-255-2763
E-mail: northeastada@cornell.edu
Website: www.ilr.cornell.edu/extension/ped/northeastADA/index.html

Region 3 (DE, DC, MD, PA, VA, WV)

DBTAC—Mid-Atlantic ADA Center
TransCen, Inc.
451 Hungerford Drive, Suite 700
Rockville, MD 20850
Phone (V/TTY): 301-217-0124
Fax: 301-217-0754
E-mail: adainfo@transcen.org
Website: www.adainfo.org

Region 4 (AL, FL, GA, KY, MS, NC, SC, TN)

DBTAC—Southeast ADA Center
Project of the Burton Blatt Institute—Syracuse University
490 Tenth Street, NW
Atlanta, GA 30318
Phone (V/TTY): 404-385-0636
Fax: 404-385-0641
E-mail: sedbtacproject@law.syr.edu
Website: www.sedbtac.org

Region 5 (IL, IN, MI, MN, OH, WI)

DBTAC—Great Lakes ADA Center
University of Illinois/Chicago
Department on Disability & Human Development
1640 West Roosevelt Road
Chicago, IL 60608
Phone (V/TTY): 312-413-1407

Fax: 312-413-1856
E-mail: gldbtac@uic.edu
website: www.adagreatlakes.org

Region 6 (AR, LA, NM, OK, TX)

DBTAC—Southwest ADA Center
Independent Living Research Utilization
2323 South Shepherd Boulevard, Suite 1000
Houston, TX 77019
Phone (V/TTY): 713-520-0232
Fax: 713-520-5785
E-mail: dlrp@ilru.org
Website: www.dlrp.org

Region 7 (IA, KS, MO, NE)

DBTAC—Great Plains ADA Center
University of Missouri/Columbia
100 Corporate Lake Drive
Columbia, MO 65203
V/TTY: 573-882-3600
Fax: 573-884-4925
E-mail: ada@missouri.edu
Website: www.adaproject.org

Region 8 (CO, MT, ND, SD, UT, WY)

DBTAC—Rocky Mountain ADA Center
Meeting the Challenge, Inc.
3630 Sinton Road, Suite 103
Colorado Springs, CO 80907
Phone (V/TTY): 719-444-0268
Fax: 719-444-0269
E-mail: technicalassistance@mtc-inc.com
Website: www.adainformation.org

Region 9 (AZ, CA, HI, NV, Pacific Basin)

DBTAC—Pacific ADA Center
555 12th Street, Suite 1030
Oakland, CA 94607-4046
Phone (V/TTY): 510-285-5600

Fax: 510-285-5614
E-mail: adatech@adapacific.org
Website: www.adapacific.org

Region 10 (AK, ID, OR, WA)

DBTAC—Northwest ADA Center
Western Washington University
6912 220th Street SW #105
Mountlake Terrace, WA 98043
Phone: 425-248-2480
Fax: 425-771-7438 (Fax)
E-mail: dbtacnw@wwu.edu
Website: www.dbtacnorthwest.org/

National Multiple Sclerosis Society

National MS Society – National Headquarters
733 Third Avenue, 3th Floor
New York, New York 10017-3288
Phone: 212-986-3240
Phone: 800-344-4867 to be directed to local chapter
www.nationalMSsociety.org

National MS Society—Denver Training and Resource Center (TRC)
700 Broadway, Suite 810
Denver, CO 80203
Phone: 303-813-1052

National MS Society—Public Policy Office
1100 New York Avenue, NW
Suite 660
Washington, DC 20005
Phone: 202-408-1500

Alabama Chapter
3840 Ridgeway Drive
Birmingham, AL 35209

Phone: 205-879-8881
E-mail: alc@nmss.org

Alaska Division—All America Chapter
511 West 41st Avenue, Suite 101
Anchorage, AK 99503
Phone: 907-562-7347
E-mail: aka@nmss.org

All America Chapter
700 Broadway, Suite 810
Denver, CO 80203
Phone: 303-813-6609

Allegheny District Chapter
1501 Reedsdale Street, Suite 105
Pittsburgh, PA 15233
Phone: 412-261-6347
E-mail: pax@nmss.org

Arizona Chapter
315 South 48th Street, Suite 101
Tempe, AZ 85281
Phone: 480-968-2488
E-mail: info@aza.nmss.org

Arkansas Division—All America Chapter
1100 N. University, Suite 255
Little Rock, AR 72207
Phone: 501-663-8104
E-mail: arr@nmss.org

Blue Ridge Chapter
One Morton Drive, Suite 106
Charlottesville, VA 22903
Phone: 434-971-8010
E-mail: vab@nmss.org

Central New England Chapter
101A First Avenue, Suite 6

Waltham, MA 02451
Phone: 781-890-4990
E-mail: communications@mam.nmss.org

Central North Carolina Chapter
2211 West Meadowview Road, Suite 30
Greensboro, NC 27407
Phone: 336-299-4136
E-mail: ncc@nmss.org

Central Pennsylvania Chapter
2040 Linglestown Road, Suite 104
Harrisburg, PA 17110
Phone: 717-652-2108
E-mail: pac@nmss.org

Central Virginia Chapter
2112 W. Laburnum Avenue, Suite 204
Richmond, VA 23227
Phone: 804-353-5008
E-mail: var@nmss.org

Colorado Chapter
700 Broadway, Suite 808
Denver, CO 80203
Phone: 303-831-0700
E-mail: general.information@coc.nmss.org

Connecticut Chapter
659 Tower Avenue, First Floor
Hartford, CT 06112
Phone: 860-714-2300
E-mail: info@ctfightsMS.org

Delaware Chapter
Two Mill Road, Suite 106
Wilmington, DE 19806
Phone: 302-655-5610
E-mail: ded@nmss.org

Eastern North Carolina Chapter
3101 Industrial Drive, Suite 210
Raleigh, NC 27609
Phone: 919-834-0678
E-mail: nct@nmss.org

Gateway Area Chapter
1867 Lackland Hill Parkway
St. Louis, MO 63146
Phone: 314-781-9020
E-mail: info@gatewaymssociety.org

Georgia Chapter
The MS Life Center
1117 Perimeter Center West, Suite E101
Atlanta, GA 30338
Phone: 404-256-9700
E-mail: mailbox@nmssga.org

Great Basin Sierra Division—All America Chapter
4600 Kietzke Lane, Suite K225
Reno, NV 89502
Phone: 775-329-7180
E-mail: nvn@nvn.nmss.org

Greater Delaware Valley Chapter
1 Reed Street, Suite 200
Philadelphia, PA 19147
Phone: 215-271-1500
E-mail: pae@nmss.org

Greater Illinois Chapter
525 West Monroe Street, Suite 900
Chicago, IL 60661
Phone: 312-421-4500
E-mail: cgic@ild.nmss.org

Greater North Jersey Chapter
1 Kalisa Way, Suite 205

Paramus, NJ 07652
Phone: 201-967-5599
E-mail: chapter@njb.nmss.org

Greater Washington Chapter
192 Nickerson Street, Suite 100
Seattle, WA 98109
Phone: 206-284-4236
E-mail: greaterWAinfo@nmsswas.org

Hampton Roads Chapter
760 Lynnhaven Parkway, Suite 201
Virginia Beach, VA 23452
Phone: 757-490-9627
E-mail: info@fightms.com

Hawaii Division —All America Chapter
418 Kuwili Street, #105
Honolulu, HI 96817
Phone: 808-532-0811
E-mail: hih@nmss.org

Idaho Division—All America Chapter
6901 W. Emerald Street, Suite 207
Boise, ID 83704
Phone: 208-388-4253
E-mail: idi@nmss.org

Indiana State Chapter
7301 Georgetown Road, Suite 112
Indianapolis, IN 46268
Phone: 317-870-2500
E-mail: fightms@msindiana.org

Inland Northwest Chapter
818 East Sharp
Spokane, WA 99202
Phone: 509-482-2022
E-mail: wai@nmss.org

Kentucky/Southeast Indiana Chapter
11700 Commonwealth Drive, Suite 500
Louisville, KY 40299
Phone: 502-451-0014
E-mail: kyw@nmss.org

Lone Star Chapter
8111 N. Stadium Drive, Suite 100
Houston, TX 77054
Phone: 713-526-8967
E-mail: txh@nmss.org

Long Island Chapter
40 Marcus Drive, Suite 100
Melville, NY 11747
Phone: 631-864-8337
E-mail: nyh@nmss.org

Louisiana Chapter
4613 Fairfield Street
Metairie, LA 70006
Phone: 504-832-4013
E-mail: louisianachapter@nmss.org

Maine Chapter
170 US Route One, Suite 200
Falmouth, ME 04105
Phone: 800-344-4867 (In State)
Phone: 800-526-8890 (Outside State)
E-mail: info@msmaine.org

Maryland Chapter
11403 Cronhill Drive, Suite E
Owings Mills, MD 21117
Phone: 443-641-1200
E-mail: info@nmss-md.org

Michigan Chapter
21311 Civic Center Drive

Southfield, MI 48076
Phone: 248-350-0020
E-mail: info@mig.nmss.org

Mid America Chapter
P. O. Box 2292
Shawnee Mission, KS 66201
Phone: 913-432-3926
E-mail: info@nmsskc.org

Mid Atlantic Chapter
9801-I Southern Pine Boulevard
Charlotte, NC 28273
Phone: 704-525-2955
E-mail: ncp@nmss.org

Mid Florida Chapter
2701 Maitland Center Parkway, Suite 100
Orlando, FL 32751
Phone: 407-478-8880
E-mail: info@flc.nmss.org

Mid Jersey Chapter
246 Monmouth Road
Oakhurst, NJ 07755
Phone: 732-660-1005
E-mail: info@njm.nmss.org

Mid South Chapter
4219 Hillsboro Road, Suite 306
Nashville, TN 37215
Phone: 615-269-9055
E-mail: tns@nmss.org

Minnesota Chapter
200 12th Avenue South
Minneapolis, MN 55415
Phone: 612-335-7900
E-mail: info@mssociety.org

Mississippi Division—All America Chapter
145 Executive Drive, Suite 1
Madison, MS 39110
Phone: 601-856-5831
E-mail: msm@nmss.org

Montana Division—All America Chapter
1629 Avenue D, Suite 2-C
Billings, MT 59102
Phone: 406-252-5927
E-mail: mtt@nmss.org

National Capital Chapter
1800 M Street, NW, Suite 750 South
Washington, DC 20036
Phone: 202-296-5363
E-mail: information@msandyou.org

Nebraska Chapter
Community Health Plaza
7101 Newport Avenue, Suite 304
Omaha, NE 68152
Phone: 402-572-3190
E-mail: nen@nmss.org

Nevada Division—All America Chapter
6000 S. Eastern Avenue, Suite 5C
Las Vegas, NV 89119
Phone: 702-736-1478
E-mail: nvl@nmss.org

New York City Chapter
733 Third Avenue, 3rd Floor
New York, NY 10017
Phone: 212-463-7787
E-mail: info@msnyc.org

North Central States Chapter
2508 S. Carolyn Avenue

Sioux Falls, SD 57106
Phone: 605-336-7017
E-mail: nth@nmss.org

North Central Texas Chapter
4086 Sandshell Drive
Fort Worth, TX 76137
Phone: 817-306-7003
E-mail: nms@nctms.org

North Florida Chapter
4237 Salisbury Road
Building #4, Suite 406
Jacksonville, FL 32216
Phone: 904-332-6810
E-mail: msnorfla@fln.nmss.org

Northern California Chapter
150 Grand Avenue
Oakland, CA 94612
Phone: 510-268-0572
E-mail: info@msconnection.org

Northwestern Ohio Chapter
401 Tomahawk Drive
Maumee, OH 43537
Phone: 419-897-9533
E-mail: nwohio@amplex.net

Ohio Buckeye Chapter
6155 Rockside Road, Suite 202
Independence, OH 44131
Phone: 800-667-7131
E-mail: webmaster@nmssoha.org

Ohio Valley Chapter
4460 Lake Forest Drive, Suite 236
Cincinnati, OH 45242
Phone: 513-769-4400
E-mail: info@ohg.nmss.org

Oklahoma Chapter
4606 East 67th Street, Building 7
Suite 103
Tulsa, OK 74136
Phone: 918-488-0882
E-mail: oke@nmss.org

Oregon Chapter
104 SW Clay Street
Portland, OR 97201
Phone: 503-223-9511
E-mail: info@defeatms.org

Pacific South Coast
5950 La Place Court, Suite 200
Carlsbad, CA 92008
Phone: 760-448-8400
E-mail: msinfo@mspacific.org

Panhandle Division—All America Chapter
6222 Canyon Drive
Amarillo, TX 79109
Phone: 806-468-8005
E-mail: txp@nmss.org

Rhode Island Chapter
205 Hallene Road, #209
Warwick, RI 02886
Phone: 401-738-8383
E-mail: rir@nmss.org

Rio Grande Division—All America Chapter
4125 Carlisle Boulevard NE, Suite A
Albuquerque, NM 87107
Phone: 505-243-2792
E-mail: nmx@nmss.org

South Central and West Kansas Division—All America Chapter
9415 E. Harry Street, Suite 706

Wichita, KS 67211
Phone: 316-264-7043
E-mail: kss@nmss.org

South Florida Chapter
3201 West Commercial Boulevard, #127
Fort Lauderdale, FL 33309
Phone: 954-731-4224
E-mail: fls@nmss.org

Southern California Chapter
2440 South Sepulveda Boulevard, Suite 115
Los Angeles, CA 90064
Phone: 310-479-4456
E-mail: ms@cal.nmss.org

Southern New York Chapter
2 Gannett Drive, Suite LC
White Plains, NY 10604
Phone: 914-694-1655
E-mail: nyv@nmss.org

Upstate New York Chapter
1650 South Avenue, Suite 100
Rochester, NY 14620
Phone: 585-271-0801
E-mail: chapter@msupstateny.org

Utah State Chapter
6364 South Highland Drive, Suite 101
Salt Lake City, UT 84121
Phone: 801-424-0113
E-mail: infoutah@nmss.org

Vermont Division—All America Chapter
75 Talcott Road, Suite 40
Williston, VT 05495
Phone: 802-864-6356
E-mail: vtn@nmss.org

West Texas Division—All America Chapter
1031 Andrews Highway, Suite 201
Midland, TX 79701
Phone: 432-522-2143
E-mail: txq@nmss.org

West Virginia Division—All America Chapter
2 Players Club Drive, Suite 104
Charleston, WV 25311
Phone: 304-343-5153
E-mail: wvt@nmss.org

Wisconsin Chapter
1120 James Drive, Suite A
Hartland, WI 53029
Phone: 262-369-4400
E-mail: info@wisms.org

Wyoming Division—All America Chapter
525 Randall Avenue, Suite 105
Cheyenne, WY 82001
Phone: 307-433-9590
E-mail: wyy@nmss.org

Assistive Technology Projects

Alabama

STAR: Alabama's Assistive Technology Resource
2125 East South Boulevard
P.O. Box 20752
Montgomery, AL 36120-0752
Executive Director: Frankie Mitchum
Phone: 334-613-3484
Phone: 800-782-7656 (In State)
Phone (TTY): 334-613-3519
Fax: 334-613-3485
E-mail: frankie.mitchum@rehab.state.al.us
Website: www.rehab.state.al.us/star

Alaska

Alaska Statewide AT Program
Department of Labor & Workforce Development
Division of Vocational Rehabilitation
801 W. 10th Street, Suite A
Juneau, AK 99801
Program Coordinator: Sean O'Brien
Phone: 800-478-4378

Phone: 907-465-6969
TTY: 907-269-3570
Fax: 907-269-3632
E-mail: sean_obrien@labor.state.ak.us
Website: www.labor.state.ak.us/at/index.htm

American Samoa

American Samoa Assistive Technology Service Project (ASATS)
Division of Vocational Rehabilitation
Department of Human Resources
Pago Pago, American Samoa 96799
Project Director: Jack Potasi
Phone: 0-11-684-699-1373
TTY: 0-11-684-233-7874
Fax: 0-11-684-699-1376
E-mail: apisap26@yahoo.com

Arizona

Arizona Technology Access Program (AzTAP)
Institute for Human Development
Northern Arizona University
2400 N. Central Avenue, Suite 300
Phoenix, AZ 85004
Director: Jill Sherman Pleasant
Phone: 602-728-9534
Phone: 800-477-9921
Fax: 602-728-9535
TTY: 602-728-9536
E-mail: jill.pleasant@nau.edu
Website: www.nau.edu/ihd/aztap/

Arkansas

Arkansas Increasing Capabilities Access Network (ICAN)
Arkansas Department of Workforce Education
Arkansas Rehabilitation Services
2201 Brookwood Drive, Suite 117
Little Rock, AR 72202
Project Director: Barry Vuletich
Phone/TTY: 501-666-8868

Phone/TTY: 800-828-2799 (In State)
Fax: 501-666-5319
E-mail: bmvuletich@ars.state.ar.us
Website: www.Arkansas-ican.org

California
California Assistive Technology Systems (CATS)
California Department of Rehabilitation
2000 Evergreen
P.O. Box 944222
Sacramento, CA 94244-2220
Project Director: Richard Devylder
Phone: 916-274-6325
TTY: 916-263-8685
Fax: 916-263-7472
E-mail: rdevylde@dor.ca.gov
Website: www.atnet.org

Colorado
Colorado Assistive Technology Program
601 E. Eighteenth Avenue, Suite 130
Denver, CO 80203
Project Director: Cathy Bodine
Phone: 303-315-1280
Phone: 800-255-3477 (In State)
TTY: 303-837-8964
Fax: 303-837-1208
E-mail: cathy.bodine@uchsc.edu
Website: www.uchsc.edu/atp/

Connecticut
Connecticut Assistive Technology Program
Department of Social Services, BRS
25 Sigourney St. 11th Floor
Hartford, CT 06106
Project Director: Dawn Lambert
Phone: 860-424-4881
Phone: 800-537-2549 (In State)
TTY: 860-424-4839

Fax: 860-424-4850
E-mail: dawn.lambert@po.state.ct.us
Website: www.CTtechact.com

Delaware

Delaware Assistive Technology Initiative (DATI)
Center for Applied Science & Engineering
University of Delaware/duPont Hospital for Children
1600 Rockland Road
P.O. Box 269
Wilmington, DE 19899-0269
Director: Beth Mineo Mollica, Ph.D.
Phone: 302-651-6790
Phone: 800-870-3284 (In State)
TTY: 302-651-6794
Fax: 302-651-6793
E-mail: dati@asel.udel.edu
Website: www.dati.org

District of Columbia

Assistive Technology Program for the District of Columbia
University Legal Services
220 I Street, NE, Suite 130
Washington, DC 20002
Program Manager: Alicia C. Johns
Phone: 202-547-0198
TTY: 202-547-2657
Fax: 202-547-2662
E-mail: ajohns@uls-dc.org
Website: www.atpdc.org

Florida

Florida Alliance for Assistive Services and Technology (FAAST Inc.)
325 John Knox Road, Bldg. 400, Suite 402
Tallahassee, FL 32303-4151
Executive Director: Jane Johnson
Phone: 888-788-9216 (In State)
Fax: 850-487-2805
TTY: 850-921-5951

E-mail: faast@faast.org
Website: www.faast.org

Georgia

Georgia Tools for Life
Georgia Department of Labor
Vocational Rehabilitation Program
Assistive Technology Unit
1700 Century Circle, Suite 300
Atlanta, GA 30345
Program Manager: Carolyn Phillips
Phone: 404-638-0384
Phone: 800-497-8665 (In State)
TTY: 404-638-3085
Fax: 404-486-0218
E-mail: info@gatfl.org
Website: www.gatfl.org

Guam

Guam System for Assistive Technology (GSAT)
University of Guam
Guam Center for Excellence in Developmental Disabilities, Education,
   Research and Service (Guam CEDDERS)
UOG Station
303 University Drive, Hse #19 Dean Circle
Mangilao, Guam 96923
Project Manager: June Quitugua
Phone: 671-735-2490
TTY: 671-735-2491
Fax: 671-734-8378
E-mail: gsat@ite.net
Website: www.uog.edu/cedders/gsat.htm

Hawaii

Assistive Technology Resource Centers of Hawaii (ATRC)
414 Kuwili Street, Suite 104
Honolulu, HI 96817
Executive Director: Barbara Fischolowitz-Leong
Phone/TTY: 808-532-7110

Phone/TTY: 800-645-3007 (In State)
Fax: 808-532-7120
E-mail: atrc@atrc.org
Website: www.atrc.org

Idaho

Idaho Assistive Technology Program
129 West Third Street
Moscow, ID 83844-4401
Project Director: Ron Seiler
Phone/TTY: 208-885-3559
Phone/TTY: 800-432-8324
Fax: 208-885-3628
E-mail: rseiler@uidaho.edu
Website: www.educ.uidaho.edu/idatech

Illinois

Illinois Assistive Technology Program
1 W. Old State Capitol Plaza, Suite 100
Springfield, IL 62701
Executive Director: Wilhelmina Gunther
Phone: 217-522-7985
Phone/TTY: 217-522-9966
Fax: 217-522-8067
E-mail: iatp@iltech.org
Website: www.iltech.org

Indiana

Assistive Technology Through Action in Indiana
Attain, Inc.
5333 Commerce Square Drive, Suite G
Indianapolis, IN 46237
Executive Director: Gary Hand
Phone: 317-543-0236
Phone: 800-528-8246 (In State)
TTY: 800-743-3333 (National)
Fax: 317-543-0237
E-mail: attain@attaininc.org
Website: www.attaininc.org

Iowa

Iowa Program for Assistive Technology
Center for Disabilities and Development
100 Hawkins Drive
Iowa City, IA 52242-1011
Director: Jane Gay
Phone: 319-353-8777
Phone: 800-779-2001 (National)
TTY: 877-686-0032
Fax: 319-384-5139
E-mail: infotech@uiowa.edu
Website: www.uiowa.edu/infotech

Kansas

Assistive Technology for Kansans Program
2601 Gabriel
Parsons, KS 67357
Project Director: Sara Sack
Phone/TTY: 620-421-8367
Phone: 800-526-3648 (In State)
Fax: 620-421-0954
E-mail: ssack@ku.edu
Website: www.atk.ku.edu

Kentucky

Kentucky Assistive Technology Service (KATS) Network
Charles McDowell Center
8412 Westport Road
Louisville, KY 40242
Director: J. Chase Forrester, J.D.
Phone: 502-429-4484
Phone: 800-327-5287 (In State)
TTY: 502-429-7116
Fax: 502-429-7114
E-mail: katsnet@iglou.com
Website: www.katsnet.org

Louisiana

Louisiana Assistive Technology Access Network (LATAN)
3042 Old Forge Road, Suite D

P.O. Box 14115
Baton Rouge, LA 70898-4115
President and CEO: Julie Nesbit
Phone/TTY: 225-925-9500
Phone/TTY: 800-270-6185 (In State)
Fax: 225-925-9560
E-mail: cpourciau@latan.org
Website: www.latan.org

Maine

Maine Consumer Information and Technology Training Exchange (CITE)
Maine CITE Coordinating Center
46 University Drive
Augusta, ME 04330
Project Director: Kathleen Powers
Phone: 207-621-3195
TTY: 207-621-3482
Fax: 207-621-3193
E-mail: kmpowers@doe.k12.me.us
Website: www.mainecite.org

Maryland

Maryland Technology Assistance Program (MDTAP)
Department of Disabilities
2301 Argonne Drive, Room T17
Baltimore, MD 21218
Executive Director: Michael Dalto
Phone/TTY: 410-554-9230
Phone/TTY: 800-832-4827 (In State)
Fax: 410-554-9237
E-mail: mdtap@mdtap.org
Website: www.mdtap.org

Massachusetts

Massachusetts Assistive Technology in Consumer's Hands (MATCH)
Massachusetts Rehabilitation Commission
27 Wormwood Street, Suite 600
Boston, MA 02110
Program Director: Karen Langley

Phone/TTY: 617-204-3600
Phone/TTY: 800-245-6543
TTY: 617-204-3868
E-mail: Karen.langley@mrc.state.ma.us
Website: www.mass.gov/mrc

Michigan
Michigan Assistive Technology Project
c/o Michigan Disability Rights Coalition
740 W. Lake Lansing Road, Suite 200
East Lansing, MI 48823
Contact: Kathryn Wakeman Wyeth
Phone/TTY: 517-333-2477
Phone: 800-760-4600 (In State)
Fax: 517-333-2677
E-mail: kdwyeth@prosynergy.org
Website: www.copower.org/AT/index.htm

Minnesota
Minnesota STAR Program
50 Sherburne Avenue, Room 309
St. Paul, MN 55155
Executive Director: Chuck Rassbach
Phone: 651-201-2640
Phone: 888-234-1267 (In-State)
TTY: 800-627-2527 (In State)
Fax: 651-282-6671
E-mail: star.program@state.mn.us
Website: www.admin.state.mn.us/assistivetechnology/

Mississippi
Mississippi Project START
P.O. Box 1698
Jackson, MS 39215-1000
Project Director: Dorothy Young
Phone: 601-987-4872
Phone/TTY: 800-852-8328 (In State)
Fax: 601-364-2349

E-mail: contactus@msprojectstart.org
Website: www.msprojectstart.org

Missouri

Missouri Assistive Technology Council
4731 South Cochise, Suite 114
Independence, MO 64055-6975
Director: Diane Golden, PhD
Phone: 816-373-5193
Phone: 800-647-8557 (In State)
TTY: 800-647-8558 (In State)
TTY: 816-373-9315
Fax: 816-373-9314
E-mail: matpmo@swbell.net
Website: www.at.mo.gov

Montana

Montana Assistive Technology Program (MATP)
Rural Institute
University of Montana
634 Eddy Avenue, CHC-009
Missoula, MT 59812
Project Director: Kathy Laurin
Phone: 406-243-5676
TTY: 877-243-5511 (In-State)
Fax: 406-243-4730
E-mail: montech@ruralinstitute.umt.edu
Website: www.montech.ruralinstitute.umt.edu

Nebraska

Nebraska Assistive Technology Partnership
5143 South 48th Street, Suite C
Lincoln, NE 68516-2204
Project Director: Mark Schultz
Phone/TTY: 402-471-0734
Phone: 888-806-6287 (In State)
Fax: 402-471-6052
E-mail: atp@atp.ne.gov
Website: www.atp.ne.gov/

Nevada

Nevada Assistive Technology Collaborative
Department of Human Resources
Office of Disability Service
3656 Research Way, Suite 32
Carson City, NV 89701
Project Administrator: Kelleen Preston
Phone: 775-687-4452
TTY: 775-687-3388
Fax: 775-687-3292
E-mail: kpreston@dhhs.nv.gov
Website: www.hr.state.nv.us/directors/disabilitysvcs/dhr_ods.htm

New Hampshire

Assistive Technology in New Hampshire (ATinNH)
University of New Hampshire
Institute on Disability/UCE
10 West Edge Drive, Suite 101
Durham, NH 03824
Project Director: Therese Willkomm
Project Coordinator: Sonke Dornblut, M.S.
Phone/TTY: 603-224-0630
Phone/TTY: 800-238-2048 (In State)
Fax: 603-228-3270
E-mail: sonke.dornblut@unh.edu
Website: www.iod.unh.edu/projects/technology_policy.html

New Jersey

Assistive Technology Advocacy Center (ATAC) of NJ P&A
New Jersey Protection and Advocacy, Inc.
210 South Broad Street, 3rd Floor
Trenton, NJ 08608
Project Director: Curtis Edmonds
Phone: 609-292-9742
Phone: 800-922-7233 (In State)
TTY: 609-633-7106
Fax: 609-777-0187
E-mail: cedmonds@njpanda.org
Website: www.njpanda.org

New Mexico

New Mexico Technology Assistance Program
435 St. Michael's Drive, Building D
Santa Fe, NM 87505
Project Director: Andrew J. Winnegar
Phone/TTY: 505-954-8533
Phone: 800-866-2253 (In State)
Fax: 505-954-8608
E-mail: AWinnegar@state.nm.us
Website: www.nmtap.com

New York

NYS Commission on Quality Care and Advocacy for Persons
  with Disabilities (CQCAPD)
401 State Street
Schenectady, NY 12305
Phone/TTY: 518-388-2888
Phone/TTY: 800-624-4143 (In State)
Fax: 518-388-2890
E-mail: webmaster@cqcapd.state.ny.us
Website: www.cqcapd.state.ny.us

North Carolina

North Carolina Assistive Technology Project
Department of Health and Human Services
Division of Vocational Rehabilitation Services
1110 Navaho Drive, Suite 101
Raleigh, NC 27609-7322
Acting Project Director: Annette Lauber
Phone/TTY: 919-850-2787
Fax: 919-850-2792
E-mail: rhiatt@ncatp.org
Website: www.ncatp.org

North Dakota

North Dakota Interagency Program For Assistive Technology (IPAT)
3509 Interstate Blvd.
Fargo, ND 58103
Project Director: Judie Lee

Phone: 701-365-4729
Phone/TTY: 800-265-4728
Fax: 701-239-7229
E-mail: jlee@polarcomm.com
Website: www.ndipat.org

Northern Mariana Islands

Commonwealth of the Northern Mariana Islands Assistive Technology Project
CNMI Council on Developmental Disabilities
Systems of Technology-Related Assistance for Individuals
  with Disabilities (STRAID)
P.O. Box 502565
Saipan, MP 96950-2565
Project Director: Tony Chong
Phone: 670-664-7000
Fax: 670-664-7030
E-mail: straid@cnmiddcouncil.org
Website: www.cnmiddcouncil.org

Ohio

Assistive Technology of Ohio
445 East Dublin Granville Road, Building L
Worthington, OH 43085
Director: William Darling
Phone/TTY: 614-293-9132
Phone/TTY: 800-784-3425 (In State)
Fax: 614-293-9127
E-mail: darling.12@osu.edu
Website: www.atohio.org

Oklahoma

Oklahoma ABLE Tech
Seretean Wellness Center
Oklahoma State University
1514 W. Hall of Fame
Stillwater, OK 74078-2026
Project Manager: Linda Jaco
Phone: 405-744-9864
Phone/TTY: 800-257-1705 (National)

Fax: 405-744-2487
E-mail: linda.jaco@okstate.edu
Website: www.okabletech.okstate.edu

Oregon

Oregon Technology Access for Life Needs Project (TALN)
Access Technologies, Inc.
3070 Lancaster Drive N.E.
Salem, OR 97305-1396
Executive Director: Laurie Brooks
Phone/TTY: 503-361-1201
Phone/TTY: 800-677-7512 (In State)
Fax: 503-370-4530
E-mail: laurie@accesstechnologiesinc.org
Website: www.accesstechnologiesinc.org

Pennsylvania

Pennsylvania's Initiative on Assistive Technology (PIAT)
Institute on Disabilities/UCEDD University Services Building
Suite 610
Temple University
1601 North Broad Street
Philadelphia, PA 19122
Program Director: Amy S. Goldman
General phone: 215-204-5966
Program Director phone: 215-204-3862
Phone/TTY: 215-204-1356
Phone: 800-204-7428 (In State)
TTY: 800-750-7428 (In State)
Fax: 215-204-9371
Program Director E-mail: piat@temple.edu
E-mail: ATinfo@temple.edu
Website: www.disabilities.temple.edu

Puerto Rico

Puerto Rico Assistive Technology Program
University of Puerto Rico
Central Administration/FILIUS Instituto
Assistive Technology Institute

Jardin Botanico Sur
1187 Calle Flamboyan
San Juan, PR 00926-1117
Program Director: Maria I. Miranda
Phone: 888-496-6035 (National)
Phone: 800-981-6033 (In Puerto Rico)
Fax: 787-754-8034
TTY: 787-767-8034
Phone: 787-764-6035
Phone: 787-764-6042
E-mail: pratp@pratp.upr.edu
Website: www.pratp.upr.edu

Rhode Island

Rhode Island Assistive Technology Access Partnership (ATAP)
Office of Rehabilitation Services
40 Fountain Street
Providence, RI 02903
Project Director: Kathleen Burrell
Phone: 401-421-7005 (Ext 326)
TTY: 401-421-7016
Fax: 401-222-3574
E-mail: kburrell@ors.ri.gov
Website: www.atap.state.ri.us

South Carolina

South Carolina Assistive Technology Program
USC School of Medicine
University Center for Excellence
Columbia, SC 29208
Project Director: Evelyn Evans
Phone/TTY: 803-935-5263
Fax: 803-935-5342
E-mail: evelyne@cdd.sc.edu
Website: www.sc.edu/scatp/

South Dakota

South Dakota Assistive Technology Program
DakotaLink

1161 Deadwood Avenue, Suite #5
Rapid City, SD 57702
Project Director: Ron Rosenboom
Phone/TTY: 605-394-6742
Phone/TTY: 800-645-0673 (In State)
Fax: 605-394-6744
E-mail: dscherer@dakotaLink.net
Website: www.DakotaLink.tie.net

Tennessee

Tennessee Technology Access Program (TTAP)
Citizens Plaza, 14th Floor
400 Deaderick Street
Nashville, TN 37248-6000
Program Director: Kevin R. Wright
Phone: 615-313-5183
Phone: 800-732-5059 (In-State)
TTY: 615-313-5695
Fax: 615-532-4685
E-mail: tn.ttap@state.tn.us
Website: www.state.tn.us/humanserv/rehab/ttap.htm

Texas

Texas Technology Access Program
Texas Center for Disability Studies
University of Texas at Austin
4030-2 West Braker Lane, Suite 220
Austin, TX 78759
Director: Penny Seay, Ph.D.
Phone: 512-232-0740
Phone: 800-828-7839 (In State)
TTY: 512-232-0762
Fax: 512-232-0761
E-mail: pseay@mail.utexas.edu
Website: www.techaccess.edb.utexas.edu

U.S. Virgin Islands

U.S. Virgin Islands Technology-Related Assistance for Individuals
  with Disabilities (TRAID)

University of the Virgin Islands/UCE
#2 John Brewers Bay
St. Thomas, U.S. VI 00801-0990
Executive Director: Yegin Habtes
Phone: 340-693-1323
Fax: 340-693-1325
E-mail: yhabtes@uvi.edu
Website: www.uvi.edu/pub-relations/VIUCEDD/index.htm

Utah
Utah Assistive Technology Program
Center for Persons With Disabilities
6855 Old Main Hill
Logan, UT 84322-6855
Program Director: Marty Blair
Phone: 435-797-3824
TTY: 435-797-7089
Fax: 435-797-2355
E-mail: uatpat@cc.usu.edu
Website: www.uatpat.org

Vermont
Vermont Assistive Technology Program
103 South Main Street
Weeks Building
Waterbury, VT 05671-2305
Project Director: Julie Tucker
Phone/TTY: 802-241-2620
Phone/TTY: 800-750-6355 (In State)
TTY: 800-241-1464
Fax: 802-241-2174
E-mail: atinfo@dail.state.vt.us
Website: www.dail.state.vt.us/atp

Virginia
Virginia Assistive Technology System (VATS)
8004 Franklin Farms Drive
P.O. Box K-300
Richmond, VA 23288-0300

Director: Ken Knorr
Phone/TTY: 804-662-9990
Phone: 800-552-5019
Fax: 804-622-9478
E-mail: ken.knorr@drs.virginia.gov
Website: www.vats.org

Washington

Washington Assistive Technology Alliance
University of Washington
Center for Technology and Disability Studies
CHDD South Building, Room 104
Box 357920
Seattle, WA 98195-7920
Project Director: Debbie Cook
Phone: 800-214-8731 (Information & Referral)
Phone: 206-685-4181
Phone/TTY: 800-841-8345 (In State)
TTY: 206-616-1396
Fax: 206-543-4799
E-mail: uwat@u.washington.edu
Website: www.wata.org

West Virginia

West Virginia Assistive Technology Systems (WVATS)
West Virginia Center for Excellence in Disabilities
Airport Research and Office Park
955 Hartman Run Road
Morgantown, WV 26505
Program Manager: Jeanne Grimm
Phone/TTY: 304-293-4692
Phone: 800-841-8436 (In State)
Fax: 304-293-7294
E-mail: jgrimm@hsc.wvu.edu
Website: www.cedwvu.org/programs/wvats

Wisconsin

Wisconsin Assistive Technology Program (WisTech)
Division of Disability and Elder Services

P.O. Box 7851
1 W. Wilson Street, Room 1151
Madison, WI 53707-7851
Program Director: Holly Laux O'Higgins
Phone: 608-266-8905
Phone/TTY: 608-267-9880
Fax: 608-267-3203
E-mail: lauxhm@dhfs.state.wi.us
Website: www.dhfs.wisconsin.gov/disabilities/wistech/index.htm

Wyoming
WIND Assistive Technology Resources (WATR), Wyoming Institute
   for Disabilities (WIND)
University of Wyoming
Box 4298
Laramie, WY 82072-4298
WATR Program Director: Sandra Root-Elledge
Phone/TTY: 307-766-2764
Phone/TTY: 800-861-4312
Fax: 307-766-2763
E-mail: watr.uw@uwyo.edu
Website: www.wind.uwyo.edu/watr

Index